THE STORYTELLING MONKEY

& The Web of Life

The Science and Practice of Awakening to Nothing

Steve Brandl

THE STORYTELLING MONKEY & The Web of Life

The Science and Practice of Awakening to Nothing

Steve Brandl

Imprint:

The information in this book is intended for educational purposes only. It does not constitute medical advice and is not a substitute for professional medical diagnosis, treatment, or care. The author is not responsible for any adverse effects resulting from the application of information contained herein. Always consult a qualified healthcare professional before making changes to your health practices.

Case studies in this book are drawn from clinical experience. Names and identifying details have been changed to protect patient privacy.

First published 2026

Publisher: Steve Brandl

Coverdesign: Steve Brandl

Foreword

"The way you are going,
is not the eternal way.
The name you are using,
is not the eternal name."
— Daodejing, Chapter 1

I need to begin with an admission. In my earlier work, particularly in Siddhartha and the Storytelling Monkey, I built a framework for understanding human consciousness that I believed was honest. I drew on neuroscience and evolutionary biology to argue that the permanent Self we call "I" is not a conscious pilot inhabiting an unconscious organism — that it is, rather, the hum of the machine itself. That when the electrical circuitry of the brain changes, the so-called permanent Self changes with it. I offered proprioception — the body's direct, pre-narrative report of the present moment — as the way out of the cage of story. What I did not do, and what I am now honest enough to acknowledge, was engage with the hardest question of all. I had heard of the hard problem of consciousness. I understood it in passing. But I was so absorbed in deconstructing the Storytelling Monkey through materialist science that I did not pause to ask what materialist science itself cannot explain: why does any of this feel like anything? Why is there something it is like to be you, reading these words, right now? Why are you not simply a biological machine processing information in the dark? No one has answered this question. Not convincingly. Not yet. And so I find myself returning to write this book — not to correct my earlier work, which I still believe is largely sound, but to take it further. To follow intellectual honesty all the way to the edge of what can be known, and then to stand there without flinching. Without filling the silence with a comfortable story. Because that silence — that gap between the neural map and the felt territory — is, I now believe, the most important territory in human experience. It is where the Storytelling Monkey runs out of road. It is where the Daodejing begins. It is where every genuine tradition of wisdom, stripped of its cultural costume, has always been pointing. In my clinical work as a Fascia-Puncture practitioner in Ho Chi Minh City, I spend my days with bodies. Not with souls or spirits or energy fields — with tissue. With the liquid matrix of connective tissue that runs from the crown of the skull to the soles of the feet, holding not just the physical structure of a person but the accumulated stories of their life.

Tight shoulders from unexpressed anger. Shortened chest muscles from years of feeling low. A chronic restriction in the lower back from a story that goes: I must hold on. There is unfinished business here. The body keeps its own records. And those records are not separate from the mind that wrote them. They are the mind, made flesh. This insight – that the division between physical and mental is itself a story, one of the Storytelling Monkey's most successful fictions – is the thread that runs through everything that follows. We are not a mind inhabiting a body, or a body accidentally generating a mind. We are one continuous, interconnected web of process. And understanding this, really understanding it – not as a concept but as a lived experience – is what this book is about. Part One deepens the science of the Storytelling Monkey, this time with the hard problem held honestly at its centre. Part Two brings the philosophy into the raw territory of a real life – my own, and those of the patients who have trusted me with their bodies and their stories. Part Three offers practice: not spiritual prescriptions, but specific, grounded techniques for quieting the Monkey without muting it entirely. Because we need it. We simply need to know what it is. Along the way, I will share wisdom from the Daodejing – which remains, for me, the most intellectually honest metaphysical framework ever articulated. And I will return again and again to the Web of Life: the fascial network that is not a metaphor for interconnection, but its literal biological reality. I hope you are ready for a deep dive into the fluid matrix of existence.

The river is already moving. We are already in it.

Let the honesty in these pages lighten your journey.

Steve Brandl

Ho Chi Minh City, Vietnam

Part One - The Monkey and the Mystery

The science of the self, and where it runs out of road

Everything that follows in this book rests on the six chapters of Part One. So before we begin, it is worth being honest about what they are and what they are not. They are not a summary of neuroscience. There are excellent books that summarise the neuroscience of consciousness, and several of them appear in the References at the back of this one. What these chapters attempt is something different: to follow the science of the Storytelling Monkey as far as it honestly goes, and then to stand, without flinching, at the point where it stops. That point is real. It is not a gap that more research will eventually fill. It is a structural feature of the territory — a place where the third-person vocabulary of science meets the first-person reality of experience, and the two cannot be made to fully coincide. The philosopher David Chalmers named it the Hard Problem of Consciousness. I think of it simply as the gate. Every genuine tradition of inquiry has stood in front of it. The honest ones admit they cannot open it. They can only point. Part One builds toward that gate. Chapter by Chapter, we lay the foundations: how the brain builds a self from prediction and pattern, why the story always arrives after the fact, how language carves the world into categories that then mistake themselves for reality, why comfort is the enemy of honest inquiry, what happens neurologically when the self temporarily dissolves, and finally — in Chapter 6 — what remains when every available scientific explanation has been taken as far as it can go. A word about a phrase you will encounter at the close of every chapter in this book: What the body knew. This is not a summary. It is an acknowledgement. The body's intelligence precedes the Monkey's narrative — the tissue holds what the mind has not yet articulated, the organism knows what the story is still working up to. In naming what the body knew, I am not concluding the chapter's argument. I am pointing at what was present before the argument began. Part One is the map. Parts Two and Three are the territory — or as close to it as words can reach. Let us begin where the Monkey begins: with a story about itself.

Chapter 1

"Without desire, one recognises the miracle. Full of desire, one recognises only the desirable."
— Daodejing, Chapter 1

The Storytelling Monkey, Revisited

Why the Brain Lies – and Why That Is Not the Whole Story

Let me start with something the previous book got right, and then something it missed: your brain did not evolve to show you the truth. It evolved to keep you alive long enough to pass on your genes. These are not the same project. In fact, they are sometimes in direct opposition. A brain optimised for survival is a brain that prioritises speed over accuracy, pattern over proof, and useful fiction over honest observation. This is what I called the Storytelling Monkey – the evolutionary software running inside the skull that generates a continuous, plausible narrative of who you are, what the world is, and what you should do next. The Monkey is not a bug. It is the most successful feature in the history of biological life on this planet. Without it, you would not be reading these words. Your ancestors who told the best stories about the rustling in the grass — There is a predator there, run — survived to reproduce. Those who waited for conclusive evidence became lunch. We are the descendants of the paranoid, the pattern-seeking, the fiction-builders. This is worth sitting with. You are not a rational being who occasionally makes emotional mistakes. You are a storytelling organism who occasionally manages to be rational. The rationality is the achievement, not the default. The story is always the first response.

The Architecture of the Monkey

In Siddhartha and the Storytelling Monkey, I drew on neuroscientist Michael Gazzaniga's split-brain research to show how the left hemisphere of the brain acts as an Interpreter — a module whose job is to construct a coherent narrative of the self, even when the actual cause of behaviour is hidden from it. The story it generates always arrives after the event. But it feels, from the inside, as if it came before. We are all doing this, every second of every day. We act on biological impulse, fascial tension, environmental trigger, and unconscious pattern — and then the Interpreter drafts the account of why 'I' chose to do that. Chapter 2 will go deeper into how this mechanism actually works. For now, the essential point is this: the Monkey is always narrating backward, and it is always convincing. Since writing that book, I have encountered a framework that deepens this insight considerably. Neuroscientist Anil Seth, in his remarkable work Being You, proposes that the brain is not a passive receiver of sensory information but a prediction machine. At every moment, the brain is generating its best model of what is likely to be happening – based on past experience, internal state, and expectation – and then comparing that model against incoming sensory data. What we experience as "reality" is not the raw data. It is the model. It is the brain's best guess, continuously updated, endlessly revised. Seth calls conscious experience "controlled hallucination." This sounds provocative, but it is precise. When two people stand in the same room, they do not experience the same room. They each experience the room their brain has predicted – shaped by memory, emotion, attention, and the particular history of the body that stands there. The room outside is the same. The room inside is always unique. Always a story. This framework explains something that puzzled me in my clinical work for years. Why do two patients with objectively similar fascial restrictions report such radically different experiences of pain? Because pain, like all experience, is not a direct readout of tissue damage. It is the brain's predictive model of threat. Change the model — change the story the nervous system is telling about the body — and the experience of pain changes with it. Sometimes dramatically. Sometimes in a single session.

The Monkey's Most Successful Story: You

Of all the stories the Monkey tells, the most persistent and the most convincing is the story of the Self. We move through life with an unquestioned conviction that there is a "pilot" behind the eyes. A permanent, coherent "I" who owns the body, directs the thoughts, and continues from moment to moment unchanged. We call this the Self, the soul, the person. And it feels absolutely real. Neuroscience tells a different story. The neurological case of Phineas Gage remains one of the most stark. In 1848, a railroad worker in Vermont survived the passage of a large iron rod through his frontal lobe. Physically, he recovered. He could speak, walk, and work. But the man was gone. Before the accident: responsible, measured, well-liked. After: impulsive, profane, unreliable. His colleagues said he was "no longer Gage."

If the Self were a permanent, non-physical entity — a soul separate from the brain — it should have remained untouched. The iron rod should have been irrelevant to the pilot. But the pilot changed completely when the hardware changed. Because the pilot is the hardware. The Self is a process running on biological circuitry. When the circuitry changes, the Self changes. There is no ghost in the machine. There is only the machine — and what it is like, from the inside, to be the machine running. Thomas Metzinger, one of the most rigorous philosophers of mind working today, proposes that what we experience as the Self is actually a "phenomenal self-model" — a representation the brain generates of itself, in order to navigate the world. The critical feature of this model is that it is transparent. We see through it rather than at it. We mistake the model for a direct window on reality. We mistake the map for the territory. Intellectual honesty — the kind that actually changes how you live, not just how you think — begins the moment you see the model as a model. Not to destroy it. You need it. But to stop being entirely at its mercy.

The Gap the Science Leaves Open

There is something the preceding framework does not account for — something I sidestepped in my earlier work, not from dishonesty but from insufficient attention. In arguing that the Self is a biological process rather than a permanent soul, I suggested – without quite saying so – that understanding the mechanism settles the matter. That once we understand the neural mechanism, we understand the phenomenon. That consciousness is explained by the hardware. It is not. There is a question that neuroscience, for all its extraordinary achievements, has not answered. Has not even come close to answering. The philosopher David Chalmers named it the Hard Problem of Consciousness, and it is this: why does any of this feel like anything? You can describe, in precise detail, every neuron firing in the visual cortex when you see the colour red. You can map every photon that strikes the retina, every electrochemical signal that travels to the brain, every region that activates in response. And when you have done all of that – when the neural story is complete – you still have not explained why red looks like something. Why there is a felt redness. Why you are not simply a biological machine processing wavelengths of light in the dark. This is not a gap that will be closed by more research. It is a structural gap – a divide between the objective, third-person description that science provides and the subjective, first-person reality of experience. No amount of information about neurons tells you what it is like to be the person who has them. I will go deeper into this in Chapter 6. For now, I want you to simply hold this: the Storytelling Monkey is real. The neuroscience is real. And there is still something that the neuroscience does not explain. Something that points beyond the map, into territory that no story can fully capture. That gap is not a failure. It is the most interesting place in human thought. It is, as the Daodejing has always known, the gate.

What the body knew:

The brain predicts before it perceives. The Self is a model, not a metaphysical entity. And somewhere between the prediction and the experience, there is a mystery that honest science has not resolved — and may never fully resolve. This is not a reason for despair. It is the beginning of genuine inquiry.

Chapter 2

"Can you let your soul embrace oneness,
and thus learn to be whole?
Can you calm the deep waters,
to reach unveiled clarity?"
— Daodejing, Chapter 10

The Hardware of the Self

What the Brain Builds, and What It Cannot Explain

Let us look more carefully at the hardware. Because if we are going to move beyond the stories the Monkey tells, we need to understand how those stories are built. Not as abstract philosophy, but as biology. As electrochemistry. As the specific, measurable activity of neurons and networks. The more precisely we understand the mechanism, the more clearly we can see both its extraordinary power and its honest limitations.

The Default Mode Network: The Monkey's Home

When neuroscientists began mapping brain activity in the 1990s, they expected to find that the brain rests when not engaged in a specific task. What they found instead was that a specific network of brain regions becomes more active during rest – actively constructing something in the absence of external demands. This is the Default Mode Network, or DMN. And what it constructs, primarily, is you. The DMN is the neural substrate of self-referential thought. It is where the brain rehearses the past – replaying conversations, reconstructing events, revising its understanding of what happened and why. It is where the brain imagines the future – anticipating threats, planning responses, constructing scenarios. And it is where the brain maintains the continuous narrative thread that makes you feel like the same person who woke up this morning, who remembers childhood, who has plans for next year. In short, the Default Mode Network is where the Storytelling Monkey lives. When the DMN is overactive – as it often is in depression, anxiety, and chronic pain – the Monkey is running without interruption, weaving an increasingly dense web of narrative identity. Past failures confirmed by present evidence. Future threats anticipated with certainty. The Self becomes rigid, defended, and convinced of its own story. When the DMN quiets – as it does in meditation, flow states, deep bodywork, and certain hypnotic states – the narrative loosens.

The Monkey falls silent. And something else becomes available: the direct experience of the present moment, before the story begins. This is not mysticism. It is functional neuroimaging data. Researchers including Judson Brewer at Brown University have shown that experienced meditators show significantly reduced DMN activity during meditation, correlated with reduced self-referential thinking and increased present-moment awareness. The data confirms what contemplative traditions have described for millennia: the quieting of the narrative self reveals something that was always there beneath it.

Gazzaniga's Interpreter: The Monkey's Press Department

Michael Gazzaniga's split-brain research remains one of the most revealing windows into how the Self is constructed. Working with patients whose corpus callosum — the bridge between left and right hemispheres — had been severed to treat severe epilepsy, Gazzaniga discovered that the two hemispheres operate with a degree of independence that is startling. In one famous experiment, the word "walk" was flashed to the right hemisphere only. The patient stood up and began to walk. When asked why, the left hemisphere — which had not seen the command — did not say "I don't know." Without hesitation, it produced a story: "I wanted to get a drink of water." The Interpreter had invented a cause. Not deliberately, not dishonestly — this is crucial. The left hemisphere was not lying. It was doing exactly what it is designed to do: generate a coherent, plausible narrative of why the organism did what it just did. It confabulated, as neurologists call it, with complete conviction and no awareness that the story was invented. We are all confabulating, all the time. The Interpreter is always running, always drafting the story of why "I" did that, said that, felt that. And the story always arrives after the event. The decision is made; the action is taken; the emotion arises — and then the Interpreter provides the account. We experience this account as memory, as intention, as will. We experience it as ourselves. Iain McGilchrist, in his extraordinary work The Master and His Emissary, argues that this left-hemisphere Interpreter doesn't just explain behaviour — it systematically replaces direct experience with a representation of itself. The right hemisphere, in McGilchrist's model, perceives the world as it is: fluid, living, relational, always in the process of becoming. The left hemisphere categorises, names, and controls — building a map of the world that is stable, manageable, and increasingly substituted for the territory it was meant to describe. The Storytelling Monkey, in this reading, is not a neutral narrator. It is a curator with an agenda: coherence, stability, and the preservation of a recognisable Self. Reality is endlessly dynamic; the Monkey's job is to make it feel fixed.

Metzinger's Transparent Self-Model

Thomas Metzinger offers perhaps the most precise philosophical account of what the Monkey is actually building. In his self-model theory of subjectivity, the brain constructs a phenomenal self-model — a representation of the organism as a whole, embedded in its environment, moving through time. The critical feature of this model is its transparency. When you look at a clean window, you don't see the glass — you see through it to whatever is on the other side. The glass is transparent. The phenomenal self-model works the same way. You don't experience it as a model. You experience it as yourself. You look through the model and take what you see to be direct reality. This transparency is why the Self feels so absolutely convincing. It is not that the Monkey has constructed a particularly good argument for the existence of a permanent I. It is that you are looking through the model without realising there is a model there at all. There is no gap, no seam, no moment where the representation reveals itself as a representation. It is seamless. It is total. It is you. Or rather: it is what you take to be you. The moment of genuine insight — what various traditions call awakening, enlightenment, or in secular terms, seeing through the illusion — is not a new belief. It is not replacing one story with a better one. It is the moment the model becomes opaque. The moment you see the glass. The moment you recognise the representation as a representation, and in that recognition, become briefly free of it. In my clinical work, I see this in the treatment room. When a patient releases a long-held fascial restriction — a pattern held in the tissue for years, sometimes decades — they sometimes experience a sudden, disorienting loosening of identity. The physical story and the psychological story release together, because they were never separate. In that moment of release, the model briefly becomes visible. Patients describe it in various ways: a sudden feeling of spaciousness, a strange lightness, a sense of not quite knowing who they are. This is not a problem to be managed. It is a glimpse of the territory.

Anil Seth's Controlled Hallucination

Anil Seth's contribution to this landscape is to bring the prediction framework – what is called predictive processing – into direct contact with the question of consciousness. His central claim is that all perception is prediction. The brain does not wait for sensory data and then process it. It continuously generates a model of what is most likely to be happening, and then compares incoming data against that model. What we experience as seeing, hearing, tasting, and feeling is the brain's best guess, continuously revised. This means that experience is always a construction. Always an interpretation. Always, in Seth's word, a hallucination – a model generated from the inside, constrained by data from the outside. The difference between a hallucination and ordinary perception, Seth suggests, is simply the degree to which the model is constrained by sensory data. In ordinary waking life, the constraint is strong. In dreaming, in psychosis, in certain meditative states, the constraint loosens and the model runs more freely. What Seth calls the "beast machine" theory extends this to the experience of the Self specifically. The most fundamental predictions the brain makes are not about the external world but about the internal state of the body.

Predictions about heartbeat, breathing, temperature, hunger — the constant background hum of the biological machine. The Self, in Seth's account, is primarily a prediction about the state of the body — an ongoing model of the organism as a whole, generated to regulate and maintain the biological processes that keep the system alive. This is why the body matters so centrally to any honest account of consciousness. The Self is not an entity that happens to inhabit a body. The Self is the body's model of itself, generated for the body's purposes, and inseparable from the body's condition. When the body changes — through illness, through injury, through the release of long-held fascial tension — the Self changes with it. Not as a secondary consequence, but as a primary expression of the same underlying process. This is what I mean when I say that the division between the physical and the psychological is a story. Not a metaphor. A literal description of the Monkey's most pervasive and most consequential fiction.

What the body knew:

The Storytelling Monkey is not a separate narrator commenting on a life that happens independently. It is built into the same biological machinery that breathes you, circulates your blood, and holds your posture. Change the tissue, and the story changes. Change the story, and the tissue changes. They are one process, perceived from different angles.

Chapter 3

"When the folk of the newly-wrought world knew beauty, then did ugliness also stir. For these are the twin strands woven into the fabric of Earth, each giving rise to its opposite."
— Daodejing, Chapter 2

The Naming Trap and the Body

How Language Carves the World – and Gets Stuck in the Tissue

Two and a half thousand years ago, Laozi opened the Daodejing with a warning that I return to more often than any other line in any other text: the way that can be spoken of is not the eternal way. The name that can be named is not the eternal name. He was not being mystical. He was being precise. Language is a system of symbols. When you look at a map of a mountain range, the ink lines on the paper are not the mountains. You cannot climb the ink. You cannot breathe the thin air of a cartographer's contour lines. The map is a useful representation of the territory – invaluable for navigation, essential for communication – but it is not the thing itself.

We understand this about paper maps. We almost never understand it about the maps we carry inside our skulls.

How Naming Stops Seeing

Watch a young child encountering a dog for the first time. Before they have the word, there is pure encounter — the smell, the warmth, the movement, the texture of fur, the sounds. A flood of raw sensory data, met with complete presence. Then someone says: dog. And the child files it. Dog. Now they know what it is. The encounter is over. The label has arrived, and with it, the illusion of understanding. From that point forward, the child sees dogs through the concept of dog. The concept is useful — it helps predict behaviour, assess threat, navigate the world. But something has been lost. The raw encounter, the direct experience of this specific, living, irreducible creature, has been replaced by a category. The territory has been traded for the map. This is the Naming Trap. And we live inside it every moment of every day. The moment we label something, we largely stop looking at it. We replace the living, shifting, infinitely complex reality with a static category. "My difficult colleague." "My bad back." "My anxious personality." "My grief." Each label is a folder into which a whole universe of experience is compressed and filed away. Useful for the Storytelling Monkey, which needs manageable categories to function. Limiting for the human being, who pays the price of never quite seeing what is actually there. The most dangerous labels are the ones we apply to ourselves. Because unlike the label "dog" — which keeps the creature at a manageable distance — the label "I am" collapses the distance entirely. When I say "I am a person with a bad back," I have done something more than describe a physical condition. I have written the condition into the story of who I am. The Monkey has incorporated the restriction into its model of the Self. And now the tissue and the narrative reinforce each other in a loop that is extraordinarily difficult to break.

Emotional Myofascial Tension: When Stories Live in the Body

In my clinical work with Fascia-Puncture, I have come to regard a concept I call Emotional Myofascial Tension — EMFT — as one of the most practically important ideas I have encountered. It is not original to me; versions of it appear in the work of Wilhelm Reich, in Peter Levine's somatic experiencing approach, in Bessel van der Kolk's research on trauma and the body. But the fascial framework gives it a specificity that I find clinically useful. The fascia — the continuous web of connective tissue, our Web of Life, that runs through every part of the body, separating, connecting, and communicating between all structures — is not a passive scaffold. It is a living, innervated, mechanically responsive tissue that adapts continuously to the forces placed upon it. Including the forces of emotion and narrative. When we experience anger and do not express it, the muscles of the shoulders, neck, and jaw contract. If the anger becomes chronic — if it is a background state rather than an acute response — those contractions become habitual. The fascia adapts to the sustained tension, thickening and shortening in response. The emotional state has been written into the tissue. The anger is no longer just a feeling; it is a posture, a restriction, a pattern in the liquid matrix of the connective web. The same is true of grief — often held as a chronic constriction across the chest, a rounding of the shoulders, a shortening of the pectoral fascia that literally pulls the body into the posture of collapse. Of fear — often held as a chronic bracing through the diaphragm and psoas, the body perpetually prepared for a threat that is no longer present. Of the unnamed, accumulated weight of a story like "I am a melancholic person" or "my body has always been difficult" — stories that the Storytelling Monkey has adopted as identity, and that the body has dutifully embodied. Antonio Damasio's somatic marker hypothesis provides the neuroscientific foundation for this observation. Damasio demonstrated, through extensive research with patients who had damage to the ventromedial prefrontal cortex, that decision-making in humans is not primarily a rational process. It is an emotional and somatic one. The brain uses the body's physiological state — the patterns of tension, arousal, and ease registered in the muscles, viscera, and fascia — as markers to guide choice and behaviour. Emotion is not a distraction from rational thought. It is the ground in which thought grows. Which means that a chronic fascial restriction is not merely a physical problem. It is a persistent somatic marker — a signal the brain is continuously reading and incorporating into its model of who you are and what the world is like. The tissue is not just storing a postural habit. It is storing a piece of the story.

One Coin, Two Sides

I want to be precise about what I am claiming here, because it is easy to misread it in either of two directions. I am not saying that physical problems are "just" psychological, or that chronic pain is a matter of wrong thinking. This is both false and cruel to the people who live with real physical suffering. The tissue is real. The restriction is real. The pain is real. Nor am I saying that psychological states are "just" physical — that depression is a chemical imbalance to be corrected with the right drug, or that grief is merely a hormonal fluctuation to be managed. This flattens the reality of human experience into something unrecognisable. What I am saying is that the division itself is the problem. Physical and psychological are not two separate domains that occasionally influence each other. They are two descriptions of one process — like the two sides of a coin. You cannot have a coin with only one side. You cannot have a body without a mind, or a mind without a body. The Storytelling Monkey that says "my back" and the tissue that holds the pattern of that story are not in a relationship. They are expressions of the same underlying reality. This is not a new insight. The Daodejing describes the universe as a system in which apparent opposites are always expressions of a deeper unity. Yin and yang are not two things; they are two aspects of one dynamic. Being and non-being arise together. The high and the low define each other. The physical and the psychological are, in this framework, exactly such a pair — apparently opposite, actually inseparable. What changes when you truly absorb this is the quality of your relationship to your own experience. When a patient comes to me with chronic shoulder tension, I do not ask: is this physical or psychological? I ask: what is being held here, and in what form? Sometimes the answer comes first from the tissue — a specific restriction pattern that points to a postural habit or old injury. Sometimes it comes from the story — a history of suppressed anger, or a narrative of needing to carry everything alone. Most often, it comes from both simultaneously. Because it always is both simultaneously. We have simply been trained to notice only one side of the coin at a time. The practice of Un-Naming — which we will explore in detail in Part Three — is the practice of learning to notice both sides at once. To feel the tension in the tissue and to hold the question of what story lives there, without rushing to an answer. To recognise the label "my difficult back" as a story, without dismissing the reality of the pain. To meet experience directly, before the Monkey has time to file it. This is harder than it sounds. The Monkey is fast. It has had a lifetime of practice. But it is possible. And when it happens – even briefly, even partially – the territory beneath the map comes into view.

What the body knew:

Every label applied to pain, emotion, or identity is a story that the Monkey has written into the tissue. Every story written into the tissue becomes a constraint on how freely the organism can move, respond, and change. Releasing the tissue and releasing the story are not two different treatments. They are two names for the same intervention.

Chapter 4

**"My mind is that of a fool — so dull am I.
The multitude are bright, while I alone am dim.
I alone am different from the others,
and I cherish this difference."**
— Daodejing, Chapter 20

The Comfort of the Lie

Why the Brain Prefers Beautiful Fictions to Uncomfortable Truths

If intellectual honesty is so liberating, why is it so rare? If the Storytelling Monkey's maps are so clearly limited — if the Self is a model, if the labels are not the things they name, if the border between physical and psychological is a fiction — why do we cling to the maps with such ferocity? Why do we feel, when someone questions our deepest stories, not curiosity but threat? The answer is neurological, evolutionary, and deeply human. Uncertainty is not merely uncomfortable. For the Storytelling Monkey, uncertainty is biological pain.

The Horror of the Open Question

The brain is a prediction machine, as we established in Chapter 1. Prediction requires a model. A model requires categories, names, and stories. When the model fails – when an event occurs that cannot be predicted, when a question arises that cannot be answered – the brain experiences something very close to physical threat. The same circuits that activate when a predator appears activate when the Monkey encounters an idea it cannot integrate into its existing story. This is why people fight, sometimes literally, to protect beliefs that have no basis in observable reality. This is why evidence that contradicts a deeply held conviction often strengthens rather than weakens it. The psychologists call this the backfire effect: challenge a core belief and the believer holds it tighter, not because the evidence is unconvincing, but because the alternative – admitting uncertainty at the level of core identity – is experienced as existential threat. The Monkey would rather be wrong and stable than honest and lost. This explains an enormous amount of human behaviour. Conspiracy theories provide a complete, internally consistent story for events that feel threatening and inexplicable. Dogmatic religion provides a fixed answer to the most terrifying questions — where did I come from, what happens when I die, is there a purpose to any of this? Political tribalism provides a clear division of the world into those who share your story and those who threaten it. All of these, from the Monkey's perspective, are preferable to the honest answer: I don't know. The dopamine hit of a story that clicks — that resolves uncertainty, that explains the unexplainable, that places the chaotic world into a manageable narrative — is real and measurable. We are literally addicted to meaning. And like all addictions, this one comes with a cost.

The Danger of the Concept Taken for Real

The most significant cost is this: when a concept is taken for reality — when the map is mistaken for the territory — the concept becomes impossible to examine or revise. Christopher Hitchens, in God is Not Great, documented with forensic precision the consequences of this mistake at the institutional level. His target was not the felt experience of transcendence, or the genuine human need for meaning and community, or the wisdom that genuine spiritual inquiry can produce. His target — and I believe he was right to make it — was the institutional insistence that a particular set of stories, written by fallible human beings in specific historical contexts, represents the absolute and unrevised truth of a universe they had barely begun to understand. The God that commands genocide, that places one tribe above all others, that punishes curiosity and rewards obedience — this is not a description of the boundless, unnameable reality that mystics across every tradition have pointed toward. This is a Storytelling Monkey's model of power, written into scripture and enforced with the considerable institutional weight of organised religion. I want to be careful here, because this is where it is easy to slide from honest critique into a different kind of dogmatism. The Monkey that says "God does not exist" with the same certainty that the Monk says "God definitely does" has simply replaced one unfounded claim with another. The honest position is neither. The honest position is this: there are real, measurable, neurologically documented states of experience in which the ordinary sense of a bounded self dissolves, in which the distinction between the individual and the universe becomes temporarily unavailable, in which something is felt that has been called, in different traditions and different languages, God, Brahman, the Dao, Nirvana, the Infinite. These states are real. The experiences are real. The transformations they can produce in a person's life are real. What is not real — or rather, what is unverifiable and therefore dishonest to claim as fact — is the interpretive story built around those experiences. The claim that the experience confirms the existence of a personal God who created the universe in six days, or who favours one group of people over all others, or who requires specific rituals of obedience and sacrifice — these are the Storytelling Monkey's additions. They are the conceptual framework applied after the fact to an experience that was, in itself, pre-conceptual. Boundless. Unnamed. The Daodejing understood this two and a half thousand years ago. "The Dao that can be named is not the eternal Dao." Not: the Dao does not exist. But: any name you give it is already a reduction. Any story you build around it is already a cage. The experience points beyond language; the institution builds a tower of language around the experience and calls the tower God.

Pseudoscience and the Same Mistake

The same error appears in the realm of what I will call comfortable pseudoscience — the use of scientific-sounding vocabulary to construct stories that provide meaning and magic without the inconvenience of rigorous testing. "Your illness is caused by blocked energy." "This crystal will align your chakras." "The universe is sending you this experience as a lesson." These are not descriptions of observable reality. They are the Storytelling Monkey generating metaphysically rich narratives to replace the honest and sometimes frightening answer: I don't fully know why this is happening, and neither does anyone else. I am not dismissive of the relief these stories can provide. A narrative that reframes suffering as meaningful can be genuinely therapeutic — and we will explore in Part Two how narrative change can produce real physiological transformation. The story does not have to be literally true to be helpful. But there is a crucial difference between using a story consciously — as a temporary scaffolding, a way of providing the Monkey with material to work with during a difficult process — and mistaking the story for reality. The first is wisdom. The second is a new cage. In my clinical practice, I encounter this distinction regularly. A patient who understands that the regression session worked because it gave the Monkey a new story to update its somatic pattern is free to continue examining, questioning, and growing. A patient who believes they literally contacted the spirit of a deceased ancestor, and builds a new metaphysical worldview on that belief, has replaced one fixed story with another. The transformation may be real in both cases. The relationship to the story is fundamentally different.

The Uncarved Block

Laozi's concept of Pu — the uncarved block — is the image I return to most often when thinking about what intellectual honesty actually requires. The uncarved block is wood before it has been shaped into anything. It contains the potential for every possible form. The moment it is carved — shaped into a table, a figure, a weapon — it becomes one thing and ceases to be all the others. The carving is a gain in specificity and a loss in possibility. Most of us spend our lives furiously carving. Carving ourselves into Success or Failure, Believer or Atheist, Healthy or Sick, Spiritual or Rational. Each carving is a story the Monkey has adopted as identity. Each story closes possibilities that the uncarved block held open. The courage to sit with the uncarved block — to tolerate the uncertainty of not yet knowing what shape you are, to resist the Monkey's urgent need to file and label and conclude — is not passivity. It is the most active thing a human being can do. Because it requires continuously overriding one of the most powerful drives in the biological system: the drive for the comfort of the story. This does not mean abandoning all stories. You need the Monkey. You need the maps. You cannot function in the world without categories, names, and narratives. The goal is not to silence the Monkey entirely — that is impossible, and the attempt produces its own distortions. The goal is to know what the Monkey is. To hold its stories lightly. To be able to put the map down, look at the territory directly, and then — with full awareness of what you are doing — pick the map back up and use it consciously. That is the practice. And it begins, as all honest practice begins, with seeing clearly what is actually happening.

What the body knew:

Comfort is not the enemy. The enemy is comfort mistaken for truth. The Monkey needs its stories, and they need not be abandoned — only seen. A story held lightly becomes a tool. A story mistaken for reality becomes a prison. The difference between the two is not in the story. It is in the quality of attention brought to it.

Chapter 5

"Look, nothing to see, call it invisible.
Listen, nothing to hear, call it soundless.
Grasp, nothing to hold, call it intangible.
Indescribility unites in oneness."
— Daodejing, Chapter 14

The Physiology of Oneness

What Happens in the Brain When the Self Dissolves

I want to tell you what it is like.
In the summer of 2022, something began to shift in my meditation practice. The experiences became deeper, more frequent, and more difficult to describe in the vocabulary available to me. I found myself reaching for language that felt inadequate — not because the experiences were vague or uncertain, but because they were more vivid, more real, than the language of ordinary experience can contain. A sense of leaving the body. Of shrinking to quantum size, or expanding to the scale of planets. Colours and shapes moving into and out of one another. A dissolving of the boundary between where I ended and the

universe began. And accompanying all of this: a quality of absolute peace. All-encompassing love. An eternity of present moment. In a note from my journal, I wrote: it feels more real than reality. I am a materialist by training and by temperament. I do not believe in souls that survive the body, or in cosmic consciousness that exists independently of the brains that briefly participate in it. But I am also intellectually honest enough to know that these experiences are real — not as metaphysical facts, but as neurological events of the first order. And they point, I believe, to something that honest science must grapple with.

Andrew Newberg and the Neurology of Transcendence

Andrew Newberg is a neuroscientist at Thomas Jefferson University in Philadelphia who has spent decades studying what happens in the brain during peak religious and meditative experiences. Using brain imaging technology, he and his colleagues have measured the neural activity of Tibetan Buddhist meditators at the peak of their practice, Franciscan nuns during intense contemplative prayer, and practitioners of various other traditions during their deepest states of communion. What they found was consistent across traditions and remarkably specific. The parietal lobes — the regions of the brain responsible for constructing the body's sense of its own boundaries in space, for maintaining the distinction between self and world, for generating the felt sense of being a located, bounded entity in a physical environment — show dramatically reduced activity during peak mystical experience. When the parietal lobes go quiet, the boundary goes with them. The felt sense of being a separate entity in a separate world dissolves. What remains — what is experienced in that dissolution — has been described in every human tradition that has systematically explored it: unity, boundlessness, the merging of self with something larger, the disappearance of the distinction between the observer and the observed. This is what the mystics have called God, or Brahman, or the Dao, or Nirvana. This is what Laozi pointed at in Chapter 14 — the thing that cannot be seen, cannot be heard, cannot be grasped, yet is unmistakably present. This is not a supernatural visitation. It is a neurological state. And it is accessible, through practice, to any human being with a brain. The term "Oneness" — which I have used in earlier work and which appears throughout the literature of contemplative experience — is, I want to be honest, slightly misleading. "One" implies a countable entity. It implies that this state is the experience of a single unified thing, as opposed to many separate things. But what meditators consistently report is not the experience of one thing. It is the experience of the dissolution of the very framework that generates the distinction between one thing and many things. It is not unity in the sense of addition — all these separate things added together to make one. It is the experience of boundlessness: the framework of separation itself is temporarily unavailable. The Daodejing does not call it one. It calls it the unnameable. Forced to describe it, Laozi calls it great. It is the state that precedes all categories — including the category of oneness.

The Flow State and the Disappearing Self

Newberg's findings converge with the research of Mihaly Csikszentmihalyi on what he called the flow state — the experience of optimal function in which self-consciousness disappears, time distorts, and performance becomes effortless. Athletes, musicians, surgeons, writers, craftspeople — all report versions of the same experience: a quality of engagement so complete that the boundary between the person and the activity dissolves. The cook in the Zhuangzi — a text I already referenced in Fascia-Puncture — embodies this state exactly.

Nourishing the Lord of Life: Excerpt from the chapter 3 of the Zhuangzi

Lord Wenhui was watching his cook carve up an ox. The cook's hands moved with a whir, his shoulders with a lurch, his feet stamped, and his knees bent - with a hiss! with a thud! - the flesh came apart as the knife sang, every movement in perfect rhythm, like the dance of the Mulberry Grove, or the chords of the Jing Shou.

"Ah, excellent!" cried Lord Wenhui. "How did you attain such skill?"

"What your servant values is the Dao, which goes beyond mere skill. When I first began to carve oxen, all I saw was the ox itself. After three years, I no longer saw the whole form, but rather the intricate structure within. And now, I move with my spirit rather than my eyes. My senses stop functioning and my spirit moves as it wills, intuitively navigating the natural spaces of the ox as I glide the knife through the great crevices and along the natural openings, never touching the slightest ligament or tendon, much less a large bone."

"A good cook changes his knife once a year because he cuts - he hacks. An average cook changes his knife once a month because he nicks - he chips. But this knife of mine has been used for nineteen years and has carved thousands of oxen, yet its blade is as sharp as if it had just come from the whetstone.

"This is because I move it through the spaces. Where there are joints, there are spaces, and the blade of my knife finds ample room. There is no congestion, no obstruction. That is why my knife remains as good as new."

"Of course, when I come to a complicated place, I see the difficulty and become cautious. My eyes focus, my movements slow, and I wield the knife with the utmost care. Then, with a subtle movement - wham! - the flesh parts like earth crumbling. Then I lift my knife and stand up, look all around, and with satisfied deliberation, wipe my knife clean and put it away."

Lord Wenhui exclaimed, "Excellent! From the words of this cook, I have learned how to nourish life!"

His knife moves through the spaces within the ox, following the natural structure without effort, without force. He does not cut; he allows. His technique has become so refined that it is no longer technique — it is direct participation in the nature of the thing. The Self has temporarily disappeared into the task. What neuroscience has found in flow states mirrors Newberg's findings in mystical states: reduced activity in the prefrontal cortex and the DMN, the quieting of the self-monitoring and narrative-generating networks. The Storytelling Monkey steps back. And in that stepping back, a different quality of engagement becomes available — one that is faster, more accurate, more fluid, and accompanied by a felt sense of rightness that ordinary self-conscious effort cannot produce. Wu Wei — the Daoist concept of effortless action, action in accordance with the natural flow of things — is not a mystical prescription. It is a description of the flow state. Of the organism functioning at its highest capacity, with the Monkey's interference temporarily suspended.

My Own Encounters with the Boundary

The meditation experiences I noted from the summer of 2022 onward were not uniform. Some sessions brought the classical light patterns — purplish at first, then brightening into blue, sometimes the felt sense of the body dissolving, of expanding beyond any boundary I could locate. Some brought visual imagery that seemed to arrive from somewhere other than deliberate thought: a figure in white at the edge of water, arms extended, radiating an unmistakable quality of love. A young child's body, seen from the inside, in a hut at the edge of an ancient forest. Some sessions were more turbulent. Anxiety. The sense of unfinished territories. Encounters with material I had not consciously been processing. What I noticed, across all of these, was a consistent relationship between the depth of the experience and the degree to which I had been able to release conceptual holding beforehand. The sessions that began with deliberate engagement with texts — with Laozi, with scripture, with philosophical frameworks — were typically shallower. The sessions that began with open presence, with what I can only describe as trusting the process before I knew what the process would bring, went deeper. The Monkey's attachment to concepts — even beautiful and true concepts — creates a kind of cognitive holding that prevents the deeper dissolution. You cannot think your way into the state that Newberg documents. Thinking is exactly what maintains the parietal activity, the DMN engagement, the narrative Self. The state is available in the gaps between thoughts. In the silence between the Monkey's sentences. One entry from my journal stays with me. I had meditated on all-encompassing love and selflessness. A very peaceful knowing arose — not a thought, exactly, but something more like a direct perception, a pre-linguistic certainty: that what we reach toward in prayer, in meditation, in the deepest moments of genuine human connection, is not separate from what we are. That the love we seek is the love we are already made of, temporarily forgotten inside the story of a separate Self. I am aware of how this sounds. I am a Fascia-Puncture practitioner who has just described something very close to what mystics have described as grace, or the presence of God. I want to be precise about what I am and am not claiming. I am not claiming that I was visited by a supernatural entity. I am not claiming that consciousness exists independently of the brain or that the boundary of the Self is illusory in any sense other than a neurological one. I am claiming that the neurological state Newberg documents — parietal quieting, DMN deactivation, the dissolution of the self-other boundary — produces an experience that is real, is transformative, and points toward something that honest science has not yet fully explained. That gap between the neural correlate and the felt experience — between the measurable brain state and what it is like, from the inside, to be in that state — is the gap we turn to in the next chapter. The hardest gap in all of human knowledge.

The Dao as the Most Honest Metaphysical Concept

Among all the frameworks I have encountered for describing the experience of boundlessness – God, Brahman, Nirvana, the Absolute, the Ground of Being – the Daodejing's Dao remains, for me, the most intellectually honest. This is not because the Dao is the correct name for whatever is encountered in the dissolution of the Self. It is because the Daodejing insists, from its very first line, that no name is correct. The Dao is explicitly and irreducibly unnameable. Any description of it is a description of something other than it – a useful pointer, not a definition. The Daodejing never claims to tell you what the Dao is. It only tells you what the Dao is not, and gestures toward the experience of directly participating in it. Chapter 25 describes something that exists before heaven and earth, without form, without sound, standing alone without changing, moving without cease, acting as the mother of all things under heaven. Forced to give it a name, Laozi calls it Great. Forced to go further, he traces the chain: humans follow earth, earth follows heaven, heaven follows the

Dao. The Dao follows what is. Itself. Nothing outside of it. No creator, no purpose, no story. Just the unceasing flow of what is.
"God confessed to me that he does not exist" — a line from my earlier work that has, I know, unsettled some readers. Let me be precise about what I meant. The God that does not exist is the God that is a person — a being with intentions, preferences, and a personality who created the universe with a plan and intervenes in history according to that plan. That God is the Storytelling Monkey's projection of human social structure onto the cosmos. It is a useful fiction for some purposes and a dangerous one for others. What does exist — what I have experienced directly, and what Newberg has documented in the brains of hundreds of practitioners — is a state in which the boundary of the individual self dissolves, and what remains feels, undeniably, like something. Something vast. Something peaceful. Something that makes the ordinary sense of a separate, anxious, striving Self feel suddenly like the small and contingent thing it actually is. Whether that something is the Dao, or a neurological artefact of parietal deactivation, or both simultaneously — that is the question we turn to next.

What the body knew:

The dissolution of the self-other boundary is not a spiritual achievement available only to the dedicated few. It is a neurological event that occurs on a spectrum — from the mild absorption of a craftsperson in their work to the profound boundlessness of deep meditative states. The parietal lobes do not distinguish between the sacred and the secular. They simply, under the right conditions, go quiet. And in that quieting, something is revealed that was always there.

Chapter 6

**"Hollowed-out clay becomes a pot;
where the clay is not, it is usable.
The usefulness of what is, lies in what is not."**
— Daodejing, Chapter 11

The Hard Problem: Standing in the Gap

Why Consciousness Cannot Be Explained Away — and Why That Matters

We have arrived at the edge of the map. Everything in the preceding chapters has been, in a sense, preparation for this moment. The Storytelling Monkey, the Default Mode Network, the transparent self-model, the controlled hallucination, the parietal quieting — all of this is the neural story. It is a remarkable story. It is, in many respects, the most sophisticated story our species has ever told about itself. But it does not answer the hardest question. How does physical process become felt experience? How does the mechanism produce the sensation?

Chalmers' Challenge

In 1995, the philosopher David Chalmers published a paper that changed the landscape of consciousness studies. It was called Facing Up to the Problem of Consciousness, and it made a distinction that philosophers and scientists have been wrestling with ever since. There are, Chalmers argued, easy problems of consciousness and hard ones. The easy problems – not easy in the sense of simple, but easy in the sense of tractable – are the problems of explaining cognitive function. How does the brain integrate information? How does attention work? How do we distinguish sleep from waking? How does the brain generate a report of its own internal states? These are difficult scientific questions, but they are questions that science knows how to address. Given enough time, enough data, enough cleverness, they will yield. The hard problem is different in kind. It is the problem of explaining how physical processes give rise to subjective experience at all – how the neural activity that we can measure in full detail produces the felt quality of being the person who has it. You are reading these words. Something is happening – photons are striking your retina, electrochemical signals are travelling to your brain, neural networks are processing the patterns and generating a representation of language and meaning. All of this is, in principle, explicable in third-person, objective, scientific terms. But there is also something it is like to be you, reading these words. There is a quality to the experience — the felt sense of the words, the particular texture of comprehension as meaning arrives, whatever emotional resonance the ideas are generating. This is the subjective, first-person reality of experience. And no amount of information about neurons, however detailed, explains why this felt quality exists. Why the physical process is accompanied by anything at all. A philosophical zombie — a being physically identical to you in every way, whose brain processes information in precisely the same way — would, in principle, behave exactly as you do. It would report that it was conscious. It would respond to pain, pursue pleasure, form memories, and make decisions. But it would have no inner life. No felt experience. No what it is like. Just the processing, in the dark. The hard problem is the question of why you are not a philosophical zombie. Why there is something it is like to be you, rather than nothing.

Three Honest Positions

Philosophers and scientists have taken three broad positions on the hard problem. Each deserves to be understood honestly, because each captures something real.

Illusionism

Illusionism — associated most closely with Daniel Dennett and Keith Frankish — argues that the hard problem is based on a mistake. There is no "what it is like." Or rather, there is, but it is itself a representation — the brain generating a model of its own states that includes the illusion of rich, qualitative experience. Frankish calls this the illusion of phenomenal consciousness. The experience of redness, of pain, of love, is real as a representational event — but the particular qualitative richness we attribute to it, the sense that there is something it is like to see red beyond the mere processing of wavelengths, is itself a confabulation of the Storytelling Monkey. This is a coherent position, and it is consistent with the materialist framework I have been building throughout this book. But it has a problem that I cannot entirely resolve: if my experience of pain is an illusion, the illusion itself still hurts. The "illusion" of what it is like seems as real, from the inside, as anything I can know.

Saying that consciousness is an illusion feels, to me, like saying that a dream is unreal – technically true in one sense, but missing something essential about the experience of dreaming.

Panpsychism

Panpsychism – associated with Philip Goff, Chalmers himself, and a growing number of philosophers – takes the opposite position. If consciousness cannot be derived from purely physical processes, then consciousness must be in some sense fundamental. Not generated by complex systems but present, in rudimentary form, at the very base of reality. Not just in humans and animals, but in some sense in everything – in the matter itself. Goff, in Galileo's Error, argues that the hard problem exists because science since Galileo has deliberately excluded consciousness from its framework. Galileo's great achievement was to create a purely quantitative science – to strip from matter all qualitative properties and describe the world entirely in terms of numbers, measurements, and mathematical relationships. This was extraordinarily productive. But it left consciousness – which is irreducibly qualitative – with no place to go. The hard problem, in

Goff's account, is the inevitable consequence of a methodology that excluded subjective experience from the start. Panpsychism has its own problems — most seriously, the so-called combination problem: how do the rudimentary "proto-conscious" properties of subatomic particles combine to produce the rich, unified experience of a human being? No one has a convincing answer.

Integrated Information Theory

Integrated Information Theory — developed by neuroscientist Giulio Tononi — takes a third path. Consciousness, in this framework, is identical with integrated information, designated by the Greek letter phi. A system is conscious to the degree that it integrates information in a way that cannot be reduced to the sum of its parts. The more integrated, the more conscious. Human brains — with their extraordinary capacity for integration across billions of neurons — have very high phi. A thermostat, which processes information but does not integrate it in any meaningful way, has virtually none. What is radical about IIT is its implication that consciousness is not localised in the brain. Any system that generates integrated information — the enteric nervous system in the gut, with its hundred million neurons; the fascial web, with its extraordinary density of mechanoreceptors and signalling molecules; the heart, with its intrinsic nervous system – participates, in some degree, in the generation of experience. The body is not a vehicle for a brain-located consciousness. The body is itself a site of experience. I find this the most interesting of the three positions, not because I am certain it is correct, but because it resonates with what I observe in the treatment room. When I release a fascial restriction in a patient's lower leg and they report, sometimes with surprise, a shift in their emotional state – a loosening of anxiety they had stopped noticing because it was so chronic, a sudden feeling of being more present in their own body – something is happening that a brain-centric account of consciousness struggles to fully explain. The tissue is not just a medium for brain signals. It is, perhaps, a participant in the generation of experience itself.

Standing in the Gap

I am not going to tell you which of these positions is correct. I do not know. No one does. The hard problem has not been solved, and I am not convinced it will be solved within any of our lifetimes. It may be that it is genuinely unsolvable

— not because we lack the intelligence or the data, but because the very tools we use to investigate the problem are themselves products of the thing we are trying to explain. To use consciousness to study consciousness is, as the philosopher says, like trying to see your own eyes without a mirror. What I want to suggest instead is that the gap itself is meaningful. That the fact of the hard problem — the stubborn, irreducible reality that there is something it is like to be a conscious organism, something that physical description does not capture — points to a dimension of existence that honest inquiry cannot simply bracket and move on from. This is where the Daodejing, for me, remains the most honest available framework. Not because it answers the question. It explicitly does not. It says the thing that can be named is not the eternal thing. It says that at the foundation of all that can be known, there is something that cannot be known — something that is, but cannot be grasped, seen, or heard. Something that is encountered not in the accumulation of information but in the dissolution of the very apparatus that accumulates it. The hard problem is not an embarrassing gap in the scientific story that will eventually be filled. It is the permanent marker of the territory's edge. It is where the map runs out. And running out is not a failure of the map. It is the map's most honest feature.

Why This Matters for Practice

You may be wondering why a book about practical transformation is spending so much time on a philosophical problem that no one has solved. The answer is this: your relationship to the hard problem changes how you practise. If you believe that consciousness is fully explained by the brain — that there is nothing more to experience than neural processing — then the practices I will describe in Part Three are sophisticated techniques for neurological self-regulation. They work because they change the brain's activity, and the brain's activity is what experience is. This is a coherent position, and the practices work on these terms. If you hold the question open — if you allow that there may be something in the felt dimension of experience that is not fully captured by the neural story — then the practices become something slightly different. Not just neurological techniques, but genuine encounters with a dimension of your own existence that you do not yet fully understand. The open question becomes, in itself, part of the practice. The willingness to not-know, to sit in the gap without filling it with a story, is the most honest form of engagement with what is actually happening. This is what I mean when I say that the Dao – the unnamed, the ungraspable, the foundation that follows only itself – is the most honest metaphysical concept available to us. It does not pretend to answer the hard problem. It insists that the hard problem cannot be answered in the terms in which it is asked. And it points, instead, toward the practice of encountering the unnameable directly – not through more thinking, more information, more story, but through the specific quality of attention that arises when the Storytelling Monkey, for once, falls silent. The experience of that silence – which I have had in meditation, which my patients have had on the treatment table, which athletes and musicians and meditators and ordinary human beings have had in the unguarded moments of genuine presence – is not the solution to the hard problem. But it is, I believe, the closest thing to a direct encounter with what the hard problem is pointing at. Something is here, feeling this, living this, reading this. Something that no story has ever quite captured, and that the silence between stories briefly reveals. That is enough to begin.

What the body knew:

The hard problem is not an obstacle to practice. It is the most honest description of why practice matters. If experience were fully explained by the brain, the felt quality of your life would be merely the readout of a biological computer. The irreducible reality of the hard problem suggests that something is here — something that participates in experience rather than merely generating it. Not as a mystical claim. As the most honest available inference from the evidence. The territory this points toward is not found at the end of more thinking. It is already present in the tissue, in the breath, in the specific quality of sensation that arises when the Monkey, for once, stops narrating what the body is doing and simply allows the body to be known.

Part Two - The Web of Life: Stories in the Flesh

Where philosophy meets lived experience Everything in Part One was argument. This is what it looks like when the argument meets a life. The chapters that follow are personal and clinical accounts — my own experiences of the Storytelling Monkey's most consequential stories, and those of the patients who have allowed me to accompany them through the release of theirs. They are not illustrations of the theory. They are evidence of a different kind: the kind that the body provides, and that no academic framework can substitute for. A word about structure. Each chapter in Part Two ends with the same phrase that closes the chapters in Part One: What the body knew. This is intentional. The body's knowledge was always ahead of the Monkey's narrative — before the story was built, the tissue was already holding what the story would later claim to explain. In naming what the body knew, I am not summarising what the chapter proved. I am acknowledging what was present before the proof began. Part Two is also where the Web of Life earns its place in the book's title. The fascial web is not a metaphor for interconnection — it is the biological reality that makes these stories possible. The tissue stores them. The tissue releases them. The Web is the medium in which every transformation in the chapters that follow actually takes place. These are stories about cages. And about what it is like when the cage opens — not from the outside, but because the story that maintained it finally changed.

Chapter 7

"When the heart is at peace,
the world is at peace.
Restraint from excessive desire
is the key to lasting abundance"
— Daodejing, Chapter 46

The Soldier, the River, and the Story That Healed Me

On Transformation, Past Lives, and What Is Actually Real

I want to tell you about the most transformative experience of my life. And then I want to take it apart, piece by piece, in front of you.

Not to diminish it. The transformation was real — I can feel it still, in my body, in how I move through the world. But the story I almost told myself about it would have been a lie. And this book is about the difference between the two.

It was the 30th of August, 2024. I was in Ho Chi Minh City, living the life I had built over a decade of clinical practice in Vietnam. I lay down for a session of Transpersonal Regression Therapy with a therapist I trusted — we will call her

Rachel. The session had a practical starting point: my chronic low back fatigue, a residue I had been carrying for years, the kind of physical tension that resists every technique because it is not purely physical. What followed in the next two hours I would not have believed if someone else had told me about it.

I. The Body Speaks First

Rachel asked me to focus on my low back. To feel it without immediately narrating it. This is harder than it sounds — the Storytelling Monkey in the skull is always ready with a label. Bad back. Old injury. Stress. But I stayed with the raw sensation. It felt like burning tight spasms. They moved — from the right low back and hip, down into the inner anterior thigh, above the right knee, medial knee, then further down into the inner ankle and the top of the foot. The spasms arrived in a sequence, like a signal travelling a line. Something was communicating through the tissue. I had seen this in hundreds of patients — the fascial web holding a pattern that the mind has long since stopped consciously noticing. The body keeps its own records. At the foot, the sensation changed. It became specific. Heavy. Like a fist-sized stone of greyish weight pressing on that precise point. And then — something shifted in the quality of the experience — it felt like a hand. A hand gripping my ankle. And it would not let go. I followed the hand upward, the way a practitioner follows a fascial line — not forcing, but listening. Lower arm. Shoulder. And then: a green uniform. A green helmet with a yellow star. Black hair. A face turned away, seen from the side. His right leg was severed at the hip. I was looking at a man who had died in battle. And he was holding my ankle. And he was not ready to go.

II. What Happened Next

I felt his emotions as though they were mine — because in that moment, inside the hypnotic state, the boundary between his experience and my experience had dissolved. A few tears moved down my cheeks without any decision from me to cry. The grief was not mine and it was completely mine, both simultaneously. What followed, guided gently by Rachel, was a process I can only describe as accompaniment. I brought him out of the battle scene. Into my apartment — an absurd, tender detail, this Vietnamese soldier in his uniform sitting in my living space. Then I returned him to the battlefield where he died, to the moment of his death from blood loss. Something in me repaired the severed leg — a gesture that made no rational sense and felt absolutely necessary. We found his wife and daughter. We said goodbye. We went to a temple on a forested hill, his preferred resting place, and then to the mass grave where he had actually been buried. I released the other souls there. I left a rainbow bridge for those not yet released. He carried a worn reddish-brown leather notebook. On its cover: the Đạo Đức Kinh – the Daodejing. I was offered a choice: to fuse with him, or to take something of his. I chose neither fusion nor nothing. I placed my left hand on his heart and my right hand on my own and took his wisdom – his capacity for letting go, of desires both physical and mental. I chose not to take his confidence, preferring to build my own. The session ended. I felt profoundly peaceful. Something in me had shifted that I could feel in my tissue the way you feel a fascial restriction release – a sudden spaciousness where there had been grip.

III. The Storytelling Monkey Steps In

Now let me do what the Storytelling Monkey desperately wanted to do the moment the session ended: build the story. The obvious narrative writes itself. A German man living in Vietnam, deeply shaped by Daoist philosophy, lies down for a regression session. He encounters a Vietnamese soldier – almost certainly from the American War, based on the uniform description – who died in battle against his will, a man who would have preferred the life of a Taoist monk on a mountain temple. This soldier was carrying the Daodejing when he died. And he chose, across whatever boundary separates the living from the dead, to attach himself to me. Because I was the one who could finally help him go. It is a beautiful story. It is precisely the kind of story the Storytelling Monkey is masterful at constructing – rich in meaning, internally consistent, emotionally resonant, cosmically just. It answers the question of why I was drawn to Vietnam, why I practice Daoist medicine, why I was carrying tension in that specific part of my body. Everything clicks together. The dopamine of meaning floods the system. There is only one problem with it. It requires me to accept claims I cannot honestly accept.

IV. *The Honest Examination*

Let me take the experience apart, not to destroy it, but to find what is actually real inside it.
The language of the experience was mine. In the hypnotic state, the brain enters a condition

similar to dreaming – the correction signal from external sensory data is reduced, and the predictive model runs with less constraint. This means the brain generates experience from its existing vocabulary. I cannot have a vision of a Vietnamese soldier in a green uniform with a yellow star unless I have previously encoded the image of such a uniform. I cannot feel the emotional texture of a man who would have preferred to be a Taoist monk unless I have already deeply inhabited Taoist philosophy. I cannot encounter a man carrying the Tao Te Ching as his most precious possession unless that book is already among the most precious things in my own inner world. The Storytelling Monkey is extraordinarily creative, but it is not a radio receiver picking up signals from the dead. It is a generative system, assembling the most meaningful available narrative from the materials it already possesses. The physical sensations were real. The burning spasms, the movement along the fascial line from low back to ankle, the sensation of pressure at the foot – these were genuine somatic experiences, not imagined. The fascial web was speaking. Something was held in that tissue. I have seen this in patients for over a decade: the body stores patterns that the mind has stopped consciously acknowledging, and under certain conditions of reduced cortical control — deep meditation, hypnosis, bodywork — those patterns surface as sensation, movement, and sometimes imagery. The transformation was real. This is the most important point, and it is where the story almost goes wrong. The transformation — the release of the tension, the peace that followed, the shift in how I related to my own desires and to the habit of holding on — was genuine and lasting. I felt it immediately in the session and I can feel its effects now. But the transformation did not happen because a Vietnamese soldier's spirit was attached to my ankle. The transformation happened because the Storytelling Monkey updated its story. The old story — held somatically as tension in the fascial web — was something like: I must hold on. There is unfinished business in this body. The new story, generated through the therapeutic process, the imagery, the emotional release, the gesture of repair and farewell, was: it is safe to let go. The letting go is the wisdom. The story changed. The physical circuit of tension broke. The release was real. The cause was narrative, not supernatural.

V. What This Teaches Us About All Transformation

This is, I believe, one of the most important insights I have encountered in years of working with bodies and philosophies simultaneously: therapeutic transformation does not require the story to be literally true. It requires the story to change. This is why prayer works for believers – not because God intervened, but because the act of prayer changes the narrative the Storytelling Monkey is running, which changes the somatic state, which changes what is possible. This is why ritual works across cultures – not because the ritual has magical properties, but because it provides the Storytelling Monkey with a structured framework for updating its story about what happened, what it means, and what comes next. This is why my regression session worked – not because I truly encountered a soldier's spirit, but because my nervous system was given a complete narrative arc: encounter, accompaniment, repair, farewell, wisdom transferred, boundary restored. The mechanism is neuroscience. The experience is real. The interpretation is the Storytelling Monkey doing what it was built to do – and in this case, it did it beautifully and helpfully. The danger is only when we mistake the story for the territory.

When we take the interpretation as literally true, we close the inquiry. We stop asking what was actually happening in the tissue, in the nervous system, in the predictive model. We trade understanding for comfort. And comfort, as we have seen throughout this book, is the cage.

VI. *Many Lives, One Web*

And yet — I want to offer you something that survives the honest examination. Something that is more beautiful than the story of a soldier's ghost, because it is true. I do have many lives. Every cell in my body was something else before it was me, and will be something else after. The carbon atoms in my hands were forged in the heart of a dying star billions of years ago. They have passed through rocks, through oceans, through countless organisms. Some of the atoms that are currently me were once part of a tree, or a river, or a human being who lived in Vietnam centuries ago. After my particular configuration of matter ceases to maintain itself, those atoms will be released back into the Web of Life — into soil, into plants, into other bodies, into the clouds above the Mekong Delta. In this sense — the only sense that survives honest scrutiny — I am indeed everywhere. I am in the stomach of a rat. I am inside a tree. I am inside the clouds. The boundary called Steve Brandl is a temporary, local, useful fiction maintained by a biological system with a powerful evolutionary interest in maintaining it. When that boundary dissolves — as it dissolves in deep meditation, in the parietal quieting that Newberg documented, in the hypnotic state, in the moment of genuine Un-Naming — what remains is not nothing. What remains is what was always there beneath the story. The boundlessness. The Dao. Not as metaphor. As physical fact. The soldier in the green uniform carrying the Tao Te Ching may not have been a literal past life. But he was, in every meaningful sense, made of the same stuff I am made of. The same carbon, the same water, the same evolutionary inheritance, the same capacity for grief and love and the desire to let go. When I felt his emotions as my own, I was not hallucinating connection. I was briefly, accurately perceiving what is always true and usually hidden: that the boundary between self and other is a story, and beneath it, there is only the one Web. That is the transformation that was real. Not that a spirit was released. But that I, for a moment, stopped believing in my own separateness. The Monkey put the book down. And I stood, unmapped, in the river.

What the body knew:

The fascial web in my lower right leg had been holding a pattern of unresolved restrictions for years. The hypnotic state allowed that pattern to surface as imagery. The imagery gave the Storytelling Monkey the narrative material it needed to update its story. The story changed. The tissue released. The transformation was somatic and psychological simultaneously — because they are not two things. They are one coin, and we have been arguing about which side is real.

Chapter 8

> **"Knowing others is intelligent;**
> **knowing yourself is wisdom.**
> **To rule over others is strength,**
> **but self-control is true power."**
> — Daodejing, Chapter 33

The Cages We Chose

A note before we begin:

This chapter describes my personal experience of releasing addictive habits. It is not a guide to addiction recovery. If you are dealing with dependency — alcohol, nicotine, substances, or anything else — please seek support from a qualified professional. The insights here may be useful alongside professional support; they are not a substitute for it.

Addiction, Habit, and the Stories That Keep Us Hooked

Transformation, I said in the previous chapter, was the single most significant experience of my life. I stand by that. And I also want to be more precise about what transformation actually is —

because the Storytelling Monkey has a very particular idea about it, and that idea is almost always wrong. The Monkey prefers transformation as event. A moment of rupture. A single session, a single revelation, a before and after with a clear line between them. This makes a satisfying story. It is also, in my experience, a fairly rare description of how actual change works. More often, transformation is accumulation. It is the slow, unannounced revision of a story that the organism has been carrying – sometimes for decades – until one day you notice, almost with surprise, that the cage you were living in is no longer locked. Sometimes it was never locked. You simply stopped checking the door. I still feel like a permanent I. Despite years of meditation, despite the regression session, despite two decades of clinical practice with the evidence of the body's plasticity in front of me every working day – the sense of a continuous self persists. This is not a failure of practice. It is the Monkey doing its job. The goal was never to destroy the Monkey. It was to see it clearly enough to choose which of its stories to keep carrying. Some of the most important awakenings in my life were not dramatic. They were the moment I noticed a cage – and realised, with something between relief and embarrassment, that I had built it myself.

The German Story

For a long time, I drank alcohol. Specifically, beer – because this is what Germans do. I accepted this story so completely that I never examined it. It was not a decision. It was the water I swam in, the air I breathed. On weekends, you drink. At social gatherings, you drink. At the end of a difficult week, especially, you drink. This is simply the shape of adult life in the culture I was raised in. I needed plenty of beer every weekend. The Monkey had incorporated this into its model of who I was – not as an addiction, which would have been an uncomfortable story, but as normalcy. As belonging. As being a functioning member of the world I had grown up in. Alongside the beer, from my teenage years: cigarettes. Most people in my environment smoked when I was growing up. The adults, the older kids, the cool ones. The story wrote itself: I am a smoker. I accepted this cage because I saw it as a door. What followed was the logic of all addiction, which is also the logic of all narrative identity: each year, a little more. Drink more, smoke more. The normal life of an adult, so I thought.

What the Body Was Saying

The body was not silent during this period. It never is. It was sending signals with considerable clarity and consistency – and I was, with equal consistency, overriding them. The thirst and the headaches after a night out. The tiredness that was not just tiredness – a particular quality of depletion, as if something essential had been taxed beyond its capacity to recover overnight. The hangovers, which are the body's honest report of what it has been asked to process. The coughing. The dizziness. The specific, unmistakable morning texture of a mouth that has spent the previous night accumulating the byproducts of heavy smoking combined with alcohol – a sensation I once heard described, accurately, as what it would feel like to have a garbage truck inside your head. I repeated this. Many times. The body sent its report. The Monkey filed it under: this is normal, this is what everyone does, the discomfort is temporary and the belonging is permanent. This is how EMFT accumulates in the addictive cycle specifically. It is not just that the tissue holds the chronic tension of stress or unexpressed emotion. The body of a chronic drinker or smoker is also holding the story that the substance is necessary – that the relaxation, the social ease, the relief from the day's weight, cannot be reached any other way. The nervous system has been trained to associate the substance with the resolution of tension. The craving is not just neurochemical. It is narrative. The dopamine cycle and the Storytelling Monkey are running the same loop: this is how relief is reached. This is who you are when you reach it.

How the Monkey Updates: Two Models

I stopped smoking gradually. The IQos device first — the same nicotine, the same ritual, but without the combustion and the tar. Then a vaporiser. Then nicotine gum, which removed the ritual entirely and left only the biochemistry. Then, one day, the gum sat in a drawer untouched, and I noticed I had not thought about it in weeks. What I did not understand at the time — though I understand it clearly now — was that I was not using willpower. I was incrementally replacing one story with another. Each step was a smaller cage than the previous one, and at each step the Monkey updated its model: this is who I am now. The final step, when it came, was not a dramatic renunciation. It was the quiet recognition that the new story — I am a non-smoker — had become more natural than the old one. The cage had dissolved not through force but through a gradual removal of the narrative architecture that maintained it.

The alcohol was different. The shift there was not incremental but something more like a sudden change in the quality of perception – not of the substance, but of the story. I took a break for four months. No dramatic resolution, no rock-bottom moment – just a decision to pause and see what the organism felt like without the weekend ritual. During those four months, something recalibrated. The tolerance that years of regular drinking had built up quietly reset. When the break ended and I returned to a drink, the gap between what alcohol felt like and what the Monkey's story had promised it would feel like became suddenly, uncomfortably visible. A few more hangovers, each one harder than the last, each one making the ratio of cost to benefit more difficult to maintain. And then – not with ceremony, not with struggle – I let the story go. I had perceived alcohol not as pleasure anymore, but as a heavy luggage I wanted to rid myself of. That shift in perception was everything. The substance had not changed. The story had.

The Neuroscience of the Cage

What I only understood fully in retrospect was that neither transition – the smoking nor the alcohol — involved willpower in any meaningful sense. Willpower is the story the Monkey tells about overcoming itself. It makes for satisfying narrative. It is also largely fiction. What actually happened, in both cases, was that the story changed. And once the story changed, the craving lost its architecture. The neuroscience is precise about this. The Default Mode Network — the Monkey's neural home, as we explored in Chapter 2 — is also the primary engine of craving. When you anticipate a drink, when you plan for it, when you feel the particular forward-lean of wanting, the DMN is running the story of what the substance will do: the ease it will bring, the particular quality of release, the sense of the day's accumulated weight finally setting down. That story generates the physiological arousal we experience as desire. The craving is not the body demanding the substance. It is the Monkey narrating the future with the substance in it — and the body responding to the narrative. This is why suppression doesn't work. Telling the Monkey not to think about the drink is telling the Monkey to run a story about not thinking about the drink. The thing you are trying to avoid is still the centre of the story. The Monkey holds it tighter. What works — what I stumbled into without knowing the neuroscience — is something closer to what this book calls Un-Naming. Not fighting the craving, but looking at it directly. Setting the label aside. Asking: what is actually here, before the Monkey calls it a need? What is almost always there, beneath the label, is something simpler. Tension. Boredom. The particular fatigue that accumulates after hours of performing a self for other people. The body's background hum of a stress that has nowhere to go. The substance was never providing something the body lacked. It was providing a story about how to reach relief — and that story was generating the biochemistry of wanting every time the familiar conditions arose. Seeing this does not dissolve the craving instantly. The neural pathways built by years of repetition do not vanish because you have understood their architecture. But seeing the architecture changes the relationship to it. The cage becomes visible. And a visible cage — as I stood in the kitchen one ordinary Tuesday, watching the thought arise and watching it pass — turns out to be considerably easier to walk out of than one you cannot see.

The Story That Was Never Quite Yours

There is one more thing I want to name, because I find it quietly liberating rather than enraging, and because the Monkey's instinct is to make it personal when it is partly structural. The stories that maintained my drinking and smoking were not generated entirely from inside my own nervous system. They arrived pre-formed from the culture I grew up in — from a Germany in which beer was woven into the social fabric as completely as bread, and from an adolescence in which smoking was the visible mark of a particular kind of belonging. I did not choose those stories any more than I chose the language I think in. The tobacco and alcohol industries invested — and continue to invest — considerable resources in ensuring those stories persist. They understand, with the precision of long practice, that the story is the product. The substance is merely the vehicle. I am not saying this to produce anger at corporations, which would be another cage. I am saying it because recognising that the narrative of a habit was partly written for you — by culture, by commerce, by the particular world you grew up inside — changes your relationship to it. It means the story was never entirely yours to begin with. And what was never fully yours is considerably easier to return. Releasing it is not a loss of identity. It is a recovery of the uncarved block.

What the body knew:

The addiction was never about the substance. It was about the story the substance belonged to – the story of belonging, of relief, of who you are when the day finally stops demanding things from you. The tissue held the tension that the story promised the substance would resolve. When the story changed, the craving lost its architecture. The cage had never been locked from the outside. It had only ever been maintained from within.

Chapter 9

**"'Nothing is softer or more yielding than water,
yet it overcomes the hard and unyielding.
This principle is understood by all,
yet practiced by few."**
— Daodejing, Chapter 78

When the Body Releases the Narrative

Five Cases from Two Decades of Clinical Practice

I write this book, in large part, because of the gap between what I know and what I can transmit. In over twenty years of clinical practice, I have watched the body's intelligence reveal itself on the treatment table — the fascial web releasing stories it has held for decades, the nervous system updating predictions it had stopped questioning, the patient's face changing in real time as something that had been fixed became, suddenly, moveable. These moments happen. Not often enough. But they happen. What I have not been able to do, in the average clinical encounter, is transmit the understanding that makes them possible. Knowledge is transmissible. I can explain myo-fascial restriction in a consultation. I can describe how the Storytelling Monkey builds its cages. I can tell a patient that the tension in their right shoulder has a narrative architecture as much as a physical one. Most of them nod. Some of them understand conceptually. Very few understand in the way that changes how they live — what the Daodejing would call knowing from the inside, the silent inner recognition that is different in kind from intellectual comprehension. This book is my longest attempt at that transmission. These cases are its evidence. They are drawn from memory — the kind of cases we do not record in patient files, because insurance companies have no column for 'story changed,' because the bureaucracy of healthcare has no code for 'the tissue released the narrative and the person was different afterward.' I have changed identifying details. The tissue is faithfully reported. A note on what these cases are not: they are not miracles, and they are not typical. Genuine transformation in clinical practice is rarer than any practitioner who cares about their work would like. Most sessions produce modest, incremental change. The cases that follow were selected precisely because they were extraordinary — moments when the conditions were right, when the tissue and the narrative released together, when something that had been held for years finally, unmistakably, let go. I offer them not as the expected outcome of Fascia-Puncture, but as illustrations of what becomes possible when the story and the body are addressed as the one coin they have always been.

CASE ONE

The Neck That Carried Everything

My first year of clinical practice. A rehabilitation centre in Germany, specialising in orthopaedic and neurological cases — inpatients, people who had exhausted the ordinary options and arrived here as a last resort before learning to live with what they carried. I was freshly graduated, a massage therapist and physical therapist who had everything to learn about what the tissue actually knows. He was sixty years old. Office work for most of his adult life, the kind of postural history that writes itself into the cervical spine over decades: forward head carriage, compressed facet joints, chronic hyperactivation of the posterior neck musculature. He had been in severe pain for months. He had seen the doctors, the physiotherapists, the specialists. He had arrived at our centre exhausted — not only by the pain, but by the accumulation of consultations that had confirmed the physical findings and left the question of relief unanswered. Each new practitioner had addressed the tissue. None of them, as far as I could tell, had addressed what the tissue was holding. I performed what we call an extension massage of the neck and shoulder region — one hand providing gentle longitudinal traction at the occiput while the other worked the paravertebral connective tissue and deep cervical fascia in long, slow strokes. The technique is not dramatic. It requires patience and a particular quality of listening through the hands. Then something happened that I had not encountered before and have encountered only rarely since. A sudden, unmistakable release — not a dramatic pop, but a quality of giving that ran through the entire posterior chain from the skull to the mid-thoracic spine. As if something that had been braced, held, maintained under continuous low-grade load, had finally received permission to stop. He stood up from the table. The pain was gone. Not reduced — gone. He stood there for a moment with the particular expression of someone who cannot quite locate something they have been carrying for so long they had stopped noticing its weight. Then his face changed entirely. In the weeks that followed, the transformation that had begun in the tissue extended into everything else. The man who had arrived miserable — Ground down by pain, by the story of a body that had stopped cooperating, by the accumulated narrative of I am someone who suffers — became, in the most literal sense I have witnessed clinically, a different person. Not a new person; the same person, with the story removed. The lightness was not performed. It was the organism returning to something it had been before the cage closed. I have thought about that case many times over the years, because it contains something important about the two available strategies for working with a story that has become a restriction. The first strategy — and the one I favour, for reasons that run through this entire book — is to drop the story entirely. Not to replace the negative narrative with a positive one, but to loosen the Monkey's grip on the narrative altogether. The lightness this patient experienced was not the result of thinking better thoughts. It was the result of the tissue releasing, the nervous system updating, the Monkey briefly losing its purchase on a story it had been running continuously. What remained was not a better story. It was the organism before the story — the uncarved block. The second strategy is the replacement of a limiting story with a more enabling one. This works, and there are clinical contexts where it is the more accessible approach. But it carries a risk the first strategy does not: a new positive story is still a story. It can become a new cage. The man who goes from I am broken to I am a healer has exchanged one fixed identity for another. The Monkey is still running. It is running a different programme. This is progress; it is not freedom. I do not offer this as a judgement. I offer it as a clinical observation from someone who has watched both strategies from the treatment table.

CASE TWO

The Woman Who Watched Someone Choose Differently

She was in her mid-forties, professionally accomplished, socially hyperactive by the standards of Ho Chi Minh City's business world — which is saying something. Her presenting complaint was sciatic nerve pain: a deep, lateral and dorsal myofascial restriction that had been producing referred pain down the right leg with the particular pattern I associate with sustained psoas tension and a Lateral Line restriction through the hip. A physical problem with a physical location. We began treating it as such. Over the course of several sessions, she mentioned, almost in passing, that her business obligations included a regular circuit of social events at which alcohol was expected, consumed, and considered more or less mandatory. The hangovers were a recurring complaint — not the primary reason she came, but present in the background of a few appointments. The tiredness, the headaches, the particular quality of the morning after a late networking dinner when the body has been given too much poison and too little sleep. She reported these with the matter-of-fact tone of someone describing the weather: this is simply what the environment produces, and one adapts. She was, in other words, inside a story so thoroughly that she could not see it from outside. The story was: this is what business people do. This is the social contract of the world I move in. Not drinking would be conspicuous, possibly insulting, certainly unusual. The hangovers were the cost of belonging.

The shift did not come from me. I offered observations about what alcohol does to fascial hydration and the vagus nerve — accurate and relevant, but not sufficient to dislodge a story that had a decade's worth of social reinforcement behind it. What dislodged it was a Muslim businessman at one of her regular evening gatherings. He was present for the full evening. He was sharp, engaged, socially at ease. He left at a reasonable hour, sober, having made better decisions than most of the other participants. He had simply not accepted the story. She described this encounter to me with something between admiration and mild disorientation — the particular cognitive register of someone encountering, for the first time as an adult, a concrete example that the story they have been living inside is optional. It had not occurred to her, in any lived sense, that the story was optional. She understood it intellectually. The Muslim businessman made it real. The transformation was gradual from that point — not a sudden conversion, but a slow revision. Her sciatica improved as the psoas, no longer maintained in chronic activation by the cortisol load of regular alcohol consumption and disrupted sleep, began to release. The myofascial restriction that had brought her to the clinic and the narrative restriction that had been framing her social life released in parallel, because they were aspects of the same underlying condition. The Web of Life does not recognise the boundary between the physical and the psychological. It simply transmits.

CASE THREE

The Woman Who Could Not Stop Talking

She ran her own business and raised three children simultaneously, which in Ho Chi Minh City's pace of life is a particular kind of endurance event. She came to me with the full catalogue: neck tension, low back pain, sciatica, heel spurs. Not one problem but the accumulated somatic residue of a life run at maximum sustained output with no systemic provision for recovery. The first thing I noticed was that she could not finish a session without her phone. The second thing I noticed was that she could not finish a sentence – or rather, could not allow me to finish mine. Before I could complete a clinical observation, a new thought had arrived that could not be held for three more seconds without being spoken. She apologised for this, which suggested she was aware of it, which suggested she had been told before. But awareness and change are different things. Her narrative, expressed in the relentless first-person singular, was: I must do this, I must do that, I am responsible for this, I am responsible for that. There was no rest in the syntax of her inner life. No pause between the obligation and the next obligation. No space in which the organism was not the active agent managing an active requirement. The Fascia-Puncture session changed this by force, in the most literal sense. Twenty minutes face-down on the treatment table with needles across the posterior meridians — the face cradle making phone use impractical, the needles making sudden movement inadvisable, the clinical environment making conversation with colleagues impossible. She called it, after the second session, forced meditation. She did not mean this as a complaint. The treatment table gave her something she had not been able to give herself: a scheduled interruption of the Monkey. Not a philosophical interruption — a structural one. The body was held in stillness by the requirements of the session. The phone was unavailable. The colleagues were absent. The Monkey, deprived of its usual external stimulation, had nowhere to go but inward. And inward, for perhaps the first time in years, it encountered quiet. The change was slow. Over months of regular sessions, the tissue released its long-held patterns — the posterior neck, the thoracolumbar fascia, the hip flexors that had been maintaining the chronic forward-lean of someone always about to begin the next task. Alongside the physical release, something else shifted. She dropped, gradually, the personal pronouns. I must became there is. My responsibility became what is needed. The Monkey's grip on the first-person singular — that most persistent of all its fictions — loosened slightly. She began to meditate between sessions. I offered recommendations; she tried several apps and found one that suited her rhythm. The treatment table had shown her that silence was available and survivable. The meditation practice maintained the access between sessions. I want to be honest about the limits of this case. She did not reach the uncarved block. Her Monkey is still running — it is simply running a somewhat quieter version of its prior programme. This is the realistic outcome of clinical work with EMFT in a busy modern life: not transformation, but loosening. Not the silencing of the narrative, but the occasional, recoverable experience of the space between the sentences. For most people in most lives, this is both the achievable and the sufficient.

CASE FOUR

The Entrepreneur Whose Colleagues Noticed First

He came to the clinic in the specific way that very busy people come: reluctantly, briefly for his regular appointment with my colleague, the chiropractor who suggested acupuncture might be good for him. He sat down with the posture of a person who has already mentally allocated ten minutes to this interaction and is managing the remaining obligations of the day in parallel.

His chief complaint was neck and shoulder tension. This is the most common presenting pattern in high-achieving urban professionals, and it tells a consistent story: sustained sympathetic activation, chronically elevated cortisol, upper trapezius and levator scapulae maintained in low-grade contraction as the postural expression of a nervous system that has not received the signal that the threat has passed. The threat, in these cases, is usually a workload. The workload, in these cases, is usually perceived as permanent. I treated his neck and shoulders with acupuncture — the standard meridian points for stress-related cervical tension, supplemented by the fascial release points I use along the posterior and lateral neck lines. The needles went in. He lay face-up. The session was forty minutes. He left. He told us later — the chiropractor relayed it — what happened when he returned to his office. His colleagues looked at him and asked what was different. Not in a vague sense: they were specific. You are so calm. You are not angry. You are concentrated in a way you usually are not.

Several of them commented independently. He had not noticed the change in himself; he was, in the most immediate sense, too inside it to see it. But the people who knew his habitual state – his baseline of compressed urgency, the low-level irritability that chronic sympathetic overactivation produces – could see the difference immediately. What interests me about this case is not the acute clinical effect, which is real and well-documented: acupuncture and fascial release do reduce sympathetic tone, do lower cortisol, do activate the vagal parasympathetic pathways. That mechanism is not in dispute. What interests me is what the observation by his colleagues produced. He heard their description of who he had been – chronically tense, not calm, not fully concentrated – and recognised it not as an external assessment but as an honest mirror. And in that recognition, a narrative became visible that had been invisible precisely because he had been living inside it: I cannot be calm. My workload does not permit calm. This level of pressure inevitably produces this level of tension. The story was not true. It had been confirmed, daily, by his own physiological state – and his own physiological state had been produced, in part, by the story. The session had broken the loop for long enough that the organism could be seen from outside it. His colleagues saw him. He saw himself through their seeing. The Monkey, briefly, encountered its own reflection. He left Vietnam shortly after our few sessions together, and I cannot report on the longer arc of his story. But the transformation was witnessed — by his colleagues, by his family, by himself. A change in one person's narrative ripples outward through everyone who lives inside the field of that person's behaviour. The stories we tell ourselves are not private. They are the air other people breathe around us. Loosening them is not a personal achievement. It is a contribution.

CASE FIVE

The Man Who Had Already Begun

He was sixty-eight years old. His medical history required more space than the standard patient file provides: three separate cancers — thyroid, bladder, bone — a benign brain tumour removed surgically, a stomach bypass to address extreme obesity. Scars on every surface. A single crutch for balance and muscle weakness that years of illness and surgery had accumulated. He moved through the world with the deliberate, considered gait of someone who has learned not to take any step for granted. The presenting complaint was headache. Not acute, not episodic – constant. A permanent baseline pain rating of six or seven on the visual analogue scale, present since the removal of the brain tumour, maintained without significant interruption for years. He had tried everything that was available to try. He was not, at this point, hopeful. But he was not without resources either. In the months before he came to me, he had found Zen practice. Not as a resolution of his situation – he was clear-eyed enough about his history to know that resolution was not a realistic frame – but as a change in his relationship to it. He had learned, through sitting practice, to observe the pain with a quality of attention that was neither suppressive nor reactive. To perceive it, in his words, as a third person would: as a phenomenon present in the field of awareness, rather than as the centre of the self. The pain remained. His relationship to the story of the pain had begun to shift. What brought him to Fascia-Puncture was not the expectation of a cure. It was, I think, curiosity – the particular openness of a person who has reached the end of expectation and found, unexpectedly, that the end of expectation is a kind of freedom. I told him, at the first appointment, that I would not offer him a treatment plan or a predicted outcome. I did not know what was possible. We would simply work, and attend to what the tissue reported, and see what emerged. The anterior, lateral, and posterior myofascial meridians of the head and neck showed the kind of dense restriction I associate with tissue that has been in sustained sympathetic activation for years – dehydrated ground substance, reduced fascial gliding, a quality of compression that the hands recognise immediately as the aftermath of chronic pain rather than acute injury. The needles, on several occasions, wound up tightly with collagen fibres as I attempted to withdraw them – a sign of both fascial engagement and the degree of dehydration in the local tissue. The web had contracted around what it was holding. Over three sessions, something shifted. The fascial release – slow, session by session, the ground substance rehydrating as the gentle mechanical stimulus of the needling encouraged fluid movement through the connective tissue – combined with what was already happening in his Zen practice. He had been observing the pain. The practice was already loosening the narrative architecture around the pain signal: the story of permanent damage, of a body irreparably diminished, of a future defined by what had been lost. The tissue release gave the nervous system a new incoming signal to compare against its predictive model. The model began to revise. Within three sessions, he experienced the first pain-free intervals he had known in years. Hours, then a day. Not consistently — the underlying pathology was genuine and complex, and I want to be careful not to present this as a clinical resolution of what it was not. But the quality of the intervals, when they came, was unmistakable. The pessimism that had been a reasonable response to an extraordinary history began, very slightly, to shift. His gait became more fluid. He recovered strength he had assumed was simply gone. He had already done the essential work before he arrived at my table. The Zen practice had changed his relationship to the story of the pain — had introduced the observing distance that prevents the Monkey's narrative from compounding the physical signal with the additional suffering of dread, of identity-as-patient, of a future seen only through what the past has taken. My contribution was the tissue work. His contribution was the narrative work he had already begun. Neither, alone, would have produced what they produced together. This is the honest account of what Fascia-Puncture can and cannot do. It can reach the tissue. It can interrupt the somatic pattern that EMFT has installed. It can create the conditions under which the nervous system's predictive model can update. What it cannot do — what no manual therapy can do — is change the story the patient brings to the table. That work belongs to the patient. The most I can do is provide a space in which the body's honest report becomes available. What the patient does with that report is always, finally, theirs.

The Neuroscience of Story-Change: What the Research Now Shows

The cases above are clinical observations from one practitioner's experience. They carry the weight of twenty years of practice and the honesty that I have tried to maintain throughout this book. They do not carry the weight of controlled trial data. What they describe, however, has now been subjected to exactly that scrutiny — and the results are worth pausing on. In 2021, a research team led by psychologist Alan Gordon and published in JAMA Psychiatry conducted a randomised controlled trial of what they call Pain Reprocessing Therapy — a structured clinical intervention built on a single core idea: that chronic pain, in many cases, is a learned brain prediction error rather than evidence of ongoing tissue damage. The tissue that originally caused the pain has healed. The brain has not updated its model. It continues to generate the pain signal because the predictive machinery has encoded the signal as necessary — as the correct response to a body that the brain still believes to be threatened. The intervention is to change the brain's relationship to its own signal. Not to suppress the pain, and not to distract from it — but to encounter it with curiosity rather than fear. To observe it, as the 68-year-old in the fifth case had already learned to do through Zen practice, without the narrative overlay that compounds the physical signal with dread, with identity, with a future written entirely in the language of what has been lost. In Gordon and Ziv's trial, sixty-six percent of participants with chronic back pain achieved pain-free or nearly pain-free status after four weeks of treatment, compared with twenty percent in the control group. These were not patients with minor discomfort. They were patients with an average of ten years of chronic pain. The mechanism was not surgical, pharmaceutical, or structural. The mechanism was narrative. The story the nervous system was telling about the body changed, and the body changed with it. This is not a new idea dressed in clinical clothing. It is the confirmation, through rigorous methodology, of what the Daodejing understood long before the age of randomised controlled trials: the soft overcomes the hard. Not by force, but by a quality of attention that the hard thing does not know how to resist. The Storytelling Monkey's pain narrative, met with the sustained, curious, non-reactive observation that Gordon and Ziv's therapy trains, loses its grip not because it has been defeated but because it has been seen. And what is seen clearly, the book of Laozi suggests, cannot maintain its power through concealment. If you are living with chronic pain — pain that has persisted beyond the expected healing period of an injury, pain that has been assessed and treated without sustained resolution — I recommend both Gordon and Ziv's book The Way Out and consultation with a practitioner trained in Pain Reprocessing Therapy. The Fascia-Puncture work described in this chapter, and the practices in Part Three, can support and complement this approach. They cannot substitute for it.

What the body knew:

The treatment table is a mirror. It shows the body what it has been holding — not through analysis, not through diagnosis, but through the direct, unhurried attention of hands that know how to listen. What the body has been holding is always both physical and narrative simultaneously, because it was always both that created it. The release, when it comes, is always both at once. The man whose neck released its decades of accumulated load did not think his way into ease. The woman who observed the Muslim businessman did not reason her way out of a story. The entrepreneur's colleagues saw something in him before he could see it in himself. The man with the headache had already begun the work. In every case, the body knew before the Monkey did. It was waiting, as it always waits, for the conditions in which the honest answer could finally emerge.

Part Three - Quieting the Monkey

The Practice of Living in the Territory

Everything in Part One was preparation. Everything in Part Two was evidence. This is where we find out what to actually do with it. Let me be honest about what Part Three is and is not. It is not a collection of techniques for achieving enlightenment. Enlightenment, as I have argued throughout this book, is not a destination — it is a quality of attention that becomes available, briefly, when the Storytelling Monkey falls silent. You cannot achieve it as you achieve a promotion or a fitness goal. The Monkey that is trying to achieve enlightenment is the Monkey. The effort is the obstacle. What Part Three offers is something more modest and more practical: a set of graduated practices for loosening the Monkey's grip. For creating the conditions under which silence becomes available. For training the organism, gradually and honestly, to spend more time in the territory and less time lost in the map. The practices move in a progression. Breathing comes first because it is always available, requires nothing, and reaches directly into the nervous system. Un-Naming deepens the practice into perception itself — learning to encounter experience before the label arrives. Myofascial work brings the practice into the tissue, where the deepest stories are stored. And the final chapter offers what all the preceding practices prepare for: the direct, repeatable encounter with the state that Newberg documented, that the Daodejing has always pointed toward, and that your own biology already knows how to enter. The sequence is a suggestion, not a prescription. Begin wherever you are drawn. Return to what genuinely opens something in you. The Monkey will have opinions about the correct way to practice. Notice that, and continue anyway.

Chapter 10

"Completely balanced, your mind emptied, follow all things and beings, in whose ascent is their return. For a moment they unfold, they flourish and blossom, then they sink back to the source. The return to the source is peace. Peace is our true nature."

— Daodejing, Chapter 16

Coming Home to the Body

Proprioception, the Web of Life, and the Pre-Narrative Now

Before there is a story, there is a sensation. Before the Storytelling Monkey can narrate your experience, the experience is already happening — in the tissue, in the fluid, in the continuous, uninterrupted report that the body sends about where it is, how it is positioned, what it is doing, and what is happening inside it at this precise moment. This report does not require language. It does not require a Storyteller to receive it. It is simply the organism knowing itself, in the most direct and immediate sense available. This is proprioception. And it is the most reliable gateway back to the territory beneath the map. What Proprioception Actually Is The word comes from the Latin proprius — one's own — and ception, perception. The perception of one's own body. In technical terms, it refers to the sensory system that informs the brain about the position and movement of body parts in space — the system that allows you to touch your nose with your eyes closed, to walk in the dark without falling, to know without looking where your hands are right now. But proprioception, properly understood, is considerably larger than this technical definition. The body's self-sensing apparatus includes mechanoreceptors distributed throughout the fascial web — sensors embedded in the connective tissue that respond to pressure, stretch, vibration, and fluid movement. It includes the interoceptive system — the sensing of the body's internal state: heartbeat, temperature, digestion, the quality of the breath. It includes the vestibular system in the inner ear, which tracks orientation and movement in space. And it includes what some researchers call the exteroceptive dimension of proprioception — the felt sense of the body's relationship to the environment immediately surrounding it. Together, these systems constitute something more than a positioning device. They constitute the body's pre-narrative report of the present moment. Before the Monkey can tell you what you are feeling, or what it means, or what you should do about it – this system is already reporting, with complete accuracy and without editorial comment, the actual state of the organism. This is what I am pointing at when I say proprioception is the foundation of the practice. Not proprioception as a technical capacity to be trained, but proprioception as a quality of listening – the practice of attending to the body's honest report before the Monkey has time to interpret it.

The Web of Life: What the Fascia Actually Is

To understand proprioception fully, you need to understand the tissue it travels through. Because the primary medium of proprioceptive information in the body is not the central nervous system – it is the fascia. The fascia is the connective tissue web that runs, without interruption, from the soles of the feet to the crown of the skull. It is not separate from the muscles, the organs, the nerves, and the bones – it surrounds them, penetrates them, and connects them into a single, continuous, tensegrity structure. Remove every organ, every muscle, every bone from the body while leaving the fascia intact, and what remains is a perfect, three-dimensional map of the body's form. The fascia is the body's shape, held in liquid. This web contains more sensory nerve endings than any other tissue in the body. The fascia is the most innervated structure in the organism – more densely populated with mechanoreceptors than muscle, more sensitive to pressure and stretch and fluid movement than almost any other tissue we have mapped. It is not passive scaffolding. It is the body's primary sensory organ. This is what I mean by the Web of Life – not a metaphor for interconnection, but the literal, biological reality of a tissue that connects everything to everything else. A restriction in the plantar fascia of the right foot creates a tensional adjustment that travels up the posterior chain to the lower back, affects the position of the sacrum, alters the mechanics of the breathing diaphragm, and influences the fascial tension around the skull. The web does not think. It does not narrate. It simply transmits – and in that transmission, every part of the organism is continuously in conversation with every other part. This is also, I want to suggest, one of the most grounded scientific bases available for the experience of interconnection that contemplative traditions have always described. When the Storytelling Monkey falls silent – when the parietal lobes go quiet and the self-other boundary dissolves — what becomes briefly perceivable is something the fascia has always known: that the boundary between inside and outside, between self and world, is a useful convention maintained by a particular level of nervous system activity. Beneath that activity, the web continues its conversation without any of the Monkey's editorial intervention.

How It Begins: Before You Were a Story

There is something I find genuinely moving about the embryological development of the fascial web, and I want to share it here because it illuminates something about proprioception that no amount of anatomy can convey directly. In the embryo, the connective tissue framework appears extraordinarily early — before the nervous system has reached anything like its adult complexity, before the organs have differentiated into their final forms, before there is anything resembling the Storytelling Monkey. The mesenchyme — the undifferentiated connective tissue from which the adult fascia develops — is the earliest architectural tissue of the body. It is the first web. It is the template upon which everything else is built. In a real sense, you were the Web of Life before you were a self. The fascial architecture preceded the neural architecture. The body's connectivity preceded the brain's capacity to narrate it. Proprioception is therefore not just a sensory system. It is a return to the organism's earliest and most fundamental mode of knowing – the direct, pre-narrative, embodied intelligence that was present before the Monkey arrived, and that will continue its quiet conversation in the tissue long after any particular story has been released. When I invite patients into proprioceptive awareness – when I ask them to simply feel where they are, without immediately narrating it – I am not asking them to learn something new. I am asking them to remember something original.

The Practice of Proprioceptive Listening

Here is where I am going to ask you to stop reading for a moment. I am sure that until you read this sentence, you have not felt your clothes since you put them on this morning. Feel them now. The weight of fabric on your shoulders. The texture against the skin of your forearms. The slight pressure of a collar, or a waistband, or socks. These sensations have been present every moment since you dressed this morning. The Monkey simply had more interesting things to narrate, and so it filtered them out. They were available the entire time. The territory was always there. This is the entry point. Not a technique, not a meditation posture, not a breathing exercise – just the simple, immediate act of attending to what the body is already reporting. From there, you can go further. Feel the surface you are sitting on – the chair or floor or cushion that has been supporting your weight all along. Notice the quality of that contact: is it hard or yielding, even or uneven? Is there more weight on one side than the other? Is the lower back in contact with the back of the chair, or floating in front of it? These are not questions to answer analytically. They are invitations to sense. And further still: try to feel the empty space around your body. Not the air as a concept, but the actual sensation – or near-sensation – of the boundary where your skin meets what is not your body. The space a few centimetres in front of your face. The space above your head. This is proprioception reaching toward its outer edge: the felt sense of the body's relationship to its immediate environment.

Listening Inside: The Body's Interior Report

Now turn the attention inward. Follow your heartbeat. Not as a concept – actually feel for the pulse. Where can you detect it? The chest is obvious, but the heartbeat is present throughout the vascular system. Can you feel it in the neck? In the wrists? In the temples, or the soles of the feet? Follow it from its source – the heart in the centre of the chest – downward through the abdomen, the pelvis, the legs, to the feet and toes. This takes patience. The Monkey will want to narrate: I can feel my pulse. Acknowledge that, and then set it aside. Stay with the actual, physical pulse – the slight, rhythmic pressure that moves through the body thirty thousand times a day without your direction or permission. From the heartbeat, shift attention to the digestive tract. Can you feel the peristaltic movements of your intestines? This is subtle – not the dramatic gurgling of acute digestion, but the background, continuous movement of the gut doing its quiet work. Most people have never attended to this. It is there. Can you feel your liver? Your pancreas? Not by reaching for anatomical knowledge – not by thinking, the liver is here, the pancreas is there – but by simply shifting awareness to those regions and waiting. Without expectation. Without the Monkey's need for a clear result. This is listening in the deepest register available without clinical equipment. What almost always happens, when people genuinely practise this, is that something shifts in the quality of their relationship to their own body. Not the dramatic release of fascial tissue, not the emotional movement of a significant EMFT discharge — something quieter. A sense of arriving somewhere that was always here. Of inhabiting the body from the inside rather than looking at it from the outside. This is what the Daodejing means by returning to the root. Not going somewhere new. Coming home to what was always present.

Moving with Proprioception: The Barefoot Principle

The practice extends naturally into movement. Walking barefoot — actually attending to the sensory information coming from the soles of the feet with each step — is one of the most direct and accessible forms of proprioceptive training available. Most of us have spent our lives wearing shoes that muffle the foot's sensory relationship with the ground. The plantar surface of the foot is one of the most densely innervated areas of the body — the fascial web of the sole connects directly to the Superficial Back Line that runs upward through the entire posterior chain. What the feet report about the ground shapes the tension pattern of the whole body. When we disconnect the feet from their sensory environment, we are disconnecting the body's most fundamental point of contact with the earth that it stands on. When you walk barefoot – slowly, attentively, in the way the Chapter 12 Un-Naming practice applies to movement – you are not just stimulating the mechanoreceptors in the sole. You are practising the direct, pre-narrative encounter with the present moment that is the foundation of every practice in this book. Each step is a sensation before it is a step. Each contact with the ground is an event in the tissue before it is a moment in a journey. Can I slow down enough to sense the contact? Can I simply arrive at where I am and how I am, without the Monkey adding a narrative to it?

Un-Naming the Body's Report

The final and most important dimension of proprioceptive practice is the quality of language – or the practice of language's suspension – that accompanies it. When the attention rests on a sensation and a label arrives – my back hurts again, my knee is tight, I'm tired – the label immediately narrows the encounter. It files the sensation under a known category and, in doing so, stops the inquiry. The Monkey has what it needs. It moves on. The practice, as we will explore in detail in Chapter 12, is to replace the personal, storied label with something more descriptive and less identified. Not my back hurts again — which incorporates the sensation into a history, a self-concept, an expectation — but there is an ache in the lower lumbar region. Not I am exhausted — but there is a quality of heaviness in the limbs, and a particular slowness in the breath. This is not a minor semantic adjustment. It is a structural shift in how the nervous system relates to what it is experiencing. The personal label activates the Default Mode Network — it becomes part of the Storytelling Monkey's ongoing narrative about who you are and what your body is like. The descriptive observation keeps the experience in the present tense, in the body, in the territory. It remains alive rather than filed. After shifting awareness to an uncomfortable area and breathing gently toward it — you might try sending a smile. This sounds, I am aware, like the kind of instruction that would make convinced materialists leave the room. But the physiology is real: a genuine, internal smile activates the facial muscles associated with positive emotional states, which sends signals through the cranial nerves that have genuine parasympathetic effects. More importantly, the quality of attention that a smile implies — curious, warm, non-combative — is the quality of attention that allows the tissue to begin releasing. You are not attacking the restriction. You are visiting it. Does the achiness change in severity when you do this? Does the sensation change in quality – from ache to pressure, from pressure to heat, from heat to something more diffuse? Does a tingling arise, or a slight numbness? Does the area feel larger or smaller than it did when you first arrived there? These questions are not seeking a particular answer. They are maintaining the quality of open, present, non-narrating attention that the tissue needs in order to release what it has been holding. The territory is speaking. Proprioception is the language. The practice is learning to listen without immediately translating. Chapter 12 will take this practice further – into the explicit Un-Naming of emotion, of self-concept, and ultimately of the observer itself. But everything in that chapter grows from the ground established here: the direct, patient, honest attention to what the body is actually reporting, before the Monkey has had time to file it under a story. The foundation is always the same. Come home to the body. It has been here the whole time.

What the body knew:

The fascial web was present before the Storytelling Monkey arrived, and it will continue its conversation after every particular story has dissolved. Proprioception is not a technique – it is the recovery of the organism's most original mode of knowing. The body does not ask what anything means. It simply reports what is. In that report – heard without interpretation, met without judgement, attended to with the patient curiosity of someone arriving home – the territory reveals itself exactly as it is.

Chapter 11

"Can you focus your breath until it becomes soft and supple, like a newborn babe?"
— Daodejing, Chapter 10

Breathing as the Bridge

The One Autonomic Function You Can Control — and Why That Changes Everything

Of all the entry points into the territory beneath the map, the breath is the most democratic. You do not need training, equipment, a quiet room, or a particular philosophical framework. You do not need to believe anything. You do not need to have read a single word of this book. The breath is already happening. It has been happening, without your permission or your awareness, since the moment you were born. The question is only whether you are going to participate in it consciously, or continue to let it run on the Monkey's autopilot. The breath is the single point of overlap between the voluntary and involuntary nervous systems. Everything else — the heartbeat, the digestive process, the regulation of hormones, the contraction of the fascia in response to emotional state — happens without your conscious involvement. You cannot decide to slow your heart rate the way you can decide to slow your breathing. You cannot choose to release the tension in your psoas the way you can choose to release the tension in your hand. But you can choose to breathe differently. And that choice ripples outward into everything the voluntary system cannot directly reach. This is not metaphor. It is anatomy.

The Vagus Nerve: The Body's Calm Highway

The autonomic nervous system — the network of nerves that regulates the body's automatic functions — operates through two primary branches. The sympathetic branch activates the stress response: heart rate accelerates, blood pressure rises, digestion pauses, the muscles brace, the fascia tightens. Every resource is redirected toward the immediate threat. This is the system that kept your ancestors alive on the savannah. It is also the system that keeps many of my patients locked in a chronic pattern of tension that their conscious minds have long since stopped noticing. The parasympathetic branch does the opposite. It is the rest-and-restore system: heart rate slows, digestion resumes, the immune system activates, the muscles soften, the fascial web hydrates and relaxes. This is the system that heals you, digests your food, consolidates your memories, and allows the deeper layers of the organism to do their quiet, essential work. The primary conduit of the parasympathetic system is the vagus nerve — the longest cranial nerve in the body, running from the brainstem through the neck, chest, and abdomen, touching the heart, lungs, liver, spleen, kidneys, and gut. Stephen Porges, whose Polyvagal Theory has transformed our understanding of how the nervous system regulates emotional and social function, describes the vagus as the body's calm highway. When it is well-toned and active, the organism is in a state of safety, openness, and connection. When it is suppressed — as it is under chronic stress, in trauma states, and in many of the patients who find their way to my treatment table — the organism is in a state of chronic activation that the Monkey happily narrates as personality: I am an anxious person. I am always tense. I have never been able to relax. Slow, deep, nasal breathing is the most direct available stimulus to the vagus nerve. When you breathe slowly and fully — when you allow the diaphragm to descend and the belly to expand on the inhale, and take your time with the exhale — you activate the vagal pathways that signal safety to the entire organism. The heart rate slows. The fascia softens. The DMN quiets. The Monkey's narrative loosens its grip. This is why the breath is the bridge. Not because breathing is spiritual — it is biological. But because the biology of conscious breathing reaches directly into the systems that the Monkey's story runs on.

Light, Slow, Deep: The Three Principles

In Fascia-Puncture, I introduced a framework for functional breathing that I summarised with the acronym LSD — Light, Slow, Deep. I want to go deeper into each principle here, because understanding why each matters changes the quality of how you practise. Light means silent. The objective is to breathe so gently that a feather placed beneath your nose would barely stir. Most people, when asked to take a deep breath, take a large, forceful breath — filling the lungs rapidly, often through the mouth, often with visible tension in the shoulders and chest. This is not functional breathing. It is the Monkey performing the idea of breathing. Gentle breathing — breathing that uses only as much air as the body actually needs — has a specific physiological effect: it allows a slight, healthy accumulation of carbon dioxide in the bloodstream. Most people believe that more oxygen is always better. In fact, oxygen delivery to the tissues depends not on the concentration of oxygen in the blood but on the balance between oxygen and carbon dioxide. The Bohr effect, named after the Danish physiologist Christian Bohr, describes how haemoglobin releases oxygen to the tissues more readily in the presence of carbon dioxide. Breathing too much — hyperventilation, even mild and chronic — reduces CO_2, constricts blood vessels, and paradoxically reduces oxygen delivery to the tissues. Light breathing optimises this balance. It makes the oxygen you already have more available. Slow means approximately six breaths per minute — an inhalation of five seconds, an exhalation of five seconds. This is the body's resonance frequency: the rhythm at which the cardiovascular, respiratory, and nervous systems synchronise most efficiently. At six breaths per minute, Heart Rate Variability — the measure of the heart's ability to flexibly adapt its rate — is maximised. High HRV is associated with resilience, emotional regulation, cognitive flexibility, and the capacity to move smoothly between states of activation and rest. Low HRV — which accompanies chronic stress and the chronic fascial tension that goes with it — is associated with rigidity, reactivity, and the kind of fixed narrative identity that the Monkey mistakes for a permanent Self. Slow breathing is, in the most literal neurological sense, the practice of flexibility. Of keeping the system responsive rather than locked. Deep does not mean large. It means directed downward – into the belly, through the full descent of the diaphragm. The diaphragm is not merely a breathing muscle. It is the roof of the body's core canister, intimately connected through fascial continuity to the pelvic floor below, the deep spinal muscles behind, and the transversus abdominis in front. It shares critical fascial connections with the psoas – the deep hip flexor that is, in my clinical experience, one of the most consistently overloaded and under-released structures in the body of a chronically stressed modern human being. When the diaphragm moves freely – when the breath is genuinely deep – it creates a rhythmic internal massage of the surrounding connective tissues. It stimulates the vagus nerve directly. It generates the intra-abdominal pressure that stabilises the spine without the chronic bracing that many people have substituted for genuine core stability. It hydrates the fascial web through the gentle pumping action of alternating pressure. Deep breathing, done correctly, is the most accessible form of self-myofascial release available. And it is happening, or can be happening, every moment of every day.

The Nose and the Now

All three of these principles – Light, Slow, Deep – are practised through the nose, exclusively. This is not a cultural preference or a yogic tradition. It is functional anatomy. The nasal passages filter, warm, and humidify incoming air in ways the mouth cannot. More significantly, nasal breathing releases nitric oxide – a molecule produced in the sinuses that has powerful vasodilatory effects, opening blood vessels and significantly improving oxygen uptake. Mouth breathing bypasses this entirely. Mouth breathing also tends to be upper-chest breathing, which activates the accessory breathing muscles of the neck and shoulders, which in turn creates or maintains fascial tension in the very areas where many people carry their chronic stress. There is one more dimension to nasal breathing that connects directly to the practice of Un-Naming, which follows in the next chapter. Breathing through the nose, with the mouth gently closed, requires a specific tongue position: the tip of the tongue resting against the hard palate, just behind the front teeth, with the body of the tongue pressing gently upward against the roof of the mouth. This position, which is the natural resting position of the tongue in a well-functioning organism, seals the oral cavity, encourages nasal breathing, and — through the fascial and muscular connections of the throat and neck — promotes vagal tone. It also, for reasons that are difficult to explain analytically but that become immediately apparent in practice, creates a quality of internal quiet. The Monkey tends to be quieter with the mouth closed and the tongue in its resting position. This is not mysticism. The motor circuits involved in speech and internal verbalisation — the Monkey's primary tool — are partially inhibited. The narrative slows. The territory becomes a little more available.

PRACTICE: *The 5:5 Foundation Practice*

Find a comfortable position — seated or lying down. Allow the eyes to close. Place one hand on the chest and one on the lower belly. Your goal: the belly hand moves, the chest hand stays still. Close the mouth gently. Rest the tongue against the roof of the mouth. Inhale slowly and lightly through the nose for a count of 5 seconds, allowing the belly to expand. Exhale slowly and completely through the nose for a count of 5 seconds, allowing the belly to soften. Continue for a minimum of 10 minutes. Twice daily if possible. When the Monkey intervenes with commentary, planning, or judgement – notice it, without engagement, and return to the count. The return is the practice. The noticing is the practice. The counting is only the scaffold.

Breathing and the Storytelling Monkey

I want to address something that many people experience when they begin a conscious breathing practice: the Monkey does not like it. The Monkey likes to be in charge. It likes to narrate, evaluate, plan, and comment. Conscious breathing – particularly slow, deliberate breathing – creates gaps in the narrative. Silence between the Monkey's sentences. And the Monkey, as we established in Chapter 4, experiences silence as threat. It will fill the gaps with restlessness, boredom, self-criticism, the sudden urgent memory of something that needs to be done, physical discomfort that seems to appear from nowhere. This is not failure. This is the practice working exactly as it should. Every moment of Monkey commentary that you notice without being swept away by is a moment of seeing the model as a model. Of standing briefly in the territory. The noticing is not a distraction from the practice. It is the practice. Over time –

and it does take time, weeks and months rather than days — the gaps lengthen. The Monkey's commentary quiets more readily. The nervous system learns, through repeated experience, that silence is safe. That the absence of a story is not the absence of the self. That the territory does not collapse when the map is folded. This is what we are working toward. Not the permanent silencing of the Monkey — which is neither possible nor desirable. But the expansion of the gaps. The growing capacity to rest, even briefly, in the space between the sentences. To be, for a moment, unmapped.

What the body knew:

The breath is not a relaxation technique. It is a direct intervention in the biological systems that the Storytelling Monkey's narrative runs on. Every slow, nasal, diaphragmatic breath is a signal to the vagus nerve that safety is available. Every moment of conscious breathing is a choice to participate in the organism's own healing capacity — to step, briefly and deliberately, out of the Monkey's story and into the body that was always already here.

Chapter 12

"True goodness is like water; it nourishes everything without asking for anything in return. Water flows into the deepest places, which others avoid."

— Daodejing, Chapter 8

Un-Naming

The Practice of Seeing Without Labels

The Naming Trap, as we explored in Chapter 3, is the Monkey's most fundamental operation. The moment an experience is labelled, it is filed. The label closes the encounter. The map replaces the territory. Un-Naming is the practice of reopening the encounter. Of learning to meet experience directly — to feel what is actually present before the Monkey can rush in with its category. It sounds simple. It is, in practice, one of the most consistently revealing things a human being can do. What makes it difficult is the same thing that makes the Naming Trap so effective: the Monkey is fast. Between the raw sensory event and the moment of conscious awareness, the brain has already run the data through its prediction model, matched it against its categories, and delivered a labelled, interpreted, storied version of experience. By the time you are aware of what you are feeling, the Monkey has already told you what it is.

Un-Naming is the practice of catching the moment before that. Or, more realistically, the practice of returning to the raw sensation after the label has arrived — of setting the label gently aside and looking again at what is actually there.

Starting With Sensation The most accessible entry point for Un-Naming is physical sensation. This is why it follows the breathing practice: the breath creates the conditions of quiet and presence that make direct sensory encounter possible. Consider pain. Pain is one of the Monkey's most elaborately labelled experiences. "My bad knee." "My old shoulder injury." "My chronic back." Each of these labels carries an entire architecture of story — a history, a prognosis, an identity, a set of expectations about what is possible and what is not. The label arrives with the sensation, and by the time the person is consciously aware of "their bad knee," they are not actually encountering their knee. They are encountering the story of their knee, which is considerably more fixed and considerably less interesting than the actual, living, dynamic tissue that is doing something real and present in this moment. Try this. Bring your attention to any area of physical discomfort or tension in your body right now. Let the label come — whatever the Monkey offers. Then, gently, set the label to one side. Not deny it. Not argue with it. Simply place it to one side, the way you might move a newspaper off a table to see what is underneath. And look at what is actually there. Is it pressure? Heat? A quality of vibration? Is there pulsing, or stillness? Is it constant, or does it shift? Is it sharp or diffuse? Is there a direction to it — something it seems to be moving toward, or away from? How large is it? Where exactly are its edges? These are not the questions of a medical diagnosis. They are the questions of direct encounter. They are the questions that treat the sensation as living territory rather than a filed case. What almost always happens when people practise this — and I have seen it consistently in patients, in my own practice, and in the accounts of practitioners across many traditions — is that the sensation changes. Not always immediately, and not always dramatically. But the relationship to it changes. The story of a permanent, fixed, chronic condition loosens slightly when the condition is encountered directly rather than through its label. The territory turns out to be more dynamic, more responsive, and more interesting than the map had suggested.

Un-Naming Emotion

The same practice applied to emotional states is simultaneously more challenging and more revealing. Emotions are the Monkey's most heavily labelled territory. "I am angry." "I am anxious." "I am sad." Each of these statements collapses a complex, shifting, embodied state into a single word — and then, critically, incorporates it into identity. I am angry. Not: there is a quality of heat and tension currently moving through my body and generating certain thoughts. I am angry. The emotion has become the Self. Un-Naming emotion does not mean denying or suppressing it. It means meeting it with the same quality of direct attention that we bring to physical sensation. Where in the body is it? What is its texture — tight or diffuse, heavy or sharp, static or moving? What is its quality as a physical experience, before the Monkey supplies the name? This is not a technique for emotional avoidance. It is, paradoxically, a technique for deeper emotional contact. When I label a state as "anxiety" and then try to manage the label, I am managing a concept. When I follow the physical reality of the state — the tightening across the chest, the contraction in the belly, the slight holding of breath, the restless quality of the hands — I am in contact with the actual experience. And from that contact, something that the Monkey's management strategy cannot produce becomes available: genuine movement. The state shifts, because it is being met rather than managed. Eugene Gendlin, the philosopher and psychotherapist who developed the Focusing technique, called this felt sense — the bodily sense of a situation before it has been put into words. He found, through decades of research into what made therapy effective, that the patients who improved most were those who could attend to this pre-verbal bodily sense — who could stay with the unclear, shifting, physical quality of an experience rather than immediately translating it into the Monkey's categories. The felt sense is the territory. The label is the map. Un-Naming is the practice of finding your way back to the territory — not to abandon the map, but to know the difference.

Un-Naming the Self

The most radical application of this practice — and the one that connects most directly to the hard problem we explored in Chapter 6, and to the dissolution of the self-other boundary that

Newberg documented — is Un-Naming the Self itself. This does not mean denying that you exist. It means, for a moment, setting aside the Monkey's ongoing narration of who you are — the history, the roles, the self-assessments, the story of your personality and your problems and your possibilities — and meeting what remains. What remains is not nothing. There is awareness here. There is sensation. There is the felt quality of being present in this body, in this moment. But the awareness that remains when the Monkey's story is temporarily suspended does not have a name. It is not a person in the way the Monkey's narrative constructs a person. It is closer to what the Daodejing points at — the uncarved block before any particular shape has been carved into it. This cannot be forced. The Monkey's attempt to achieve self-un-naming is the Monkey doing what the Monkey does — generating a story about the absence of story. The Un-Naming of the Self tends to arrive as a side effect of the other practices, when the nervous system has quieted enough and the breath has steadied enough and the attention has practised enough that the Monkey's narrative simply slows, and in that slowing, something is briefly, quietly available that the narrative had been obscuring. Do not aim for it. Practice the foundations. The silence opens on its own.

PRACTICE: ***The Un-Naming Practice – Three Stages***

STAGE 1 – SENSATION (5 minutes): Begin with the breathing practice. Then bring attention to any physical sensation in the body. When the label arrives ('tension,' 'pain,' 'tightness'), acknowledge it and set it gently aside. Ask instead: what is the raw quality of what is here? Pressure, heat, vibration, pulse, stillness? Stay with the actual sensation for as long as you can before the Monkey re-labels it. When it re-labels, set the label aside again. Return. This is the practice.

STAGE 2 – EMOTION (5 minutes): Bring attention to your emotional state right now. Let the label come. Then ask: where in the body is this? What is its physical texture? Follow it as a sensation rather than a concept. Notice whether the state shifts when it is met directly rather than managed through its label.

STAGE 3 – OBSERVER (5 minutes): Ask, gently: who is noticing all of this? Do not answer in words. Simply rest in the question itself, and notice what is there before the Monkey supplies an answer. This is not a philosophical exercise. It is a direct inquiry. The answer, if it arrives at all, will not be a concept. It will be a quality of presence that precedes all the Monkey's categories.

A note: these stages are not rigid. Some days Stage 1 absorbs the entire session. This is not failure. The territory of sensation is inexhaustible.

Un-Naming in Daily Life

The practice does not end with the formal session. In fact, the formal session is only the training ground for the real practice: bringing Un-Naming into the texture of ordinary daily life. Every moment of direct sensory encounter — tasting food without immediately evaluating it, listening to a person without already constructing your response, feeling the contact of your feet with the ground as you walk rather than thinking about where you are going — is an act of Un-Naming. Every moment you catch the Monkey labelling and choose to stay with the raw experience for one breath longer is a moment of territory rather than map. These moments accumulate. The nervous system learns that direct encounter is safe. The Monkey learns that it does not need to name everything instantly. The gaps between the sentences widen. And in those gaps, the river flows.

What the body knew:

The label is not the enemy. The label is the Monkey's gift — the tool that makes navigation possible. But the label is not the thing. Between the sensation and the name, there is a moment of pure encounter that the practice of Un-Naming is designed to lengthen. In that moment, the body is already practising what the mind is still learning to allow.

Chapter 13

"Living beings are soft and yielding; dead things are hard and rigid. Thus, hardness and rigidity are associated with death, while softness and flexibility are associated with life."

— Daodejing, Chapter 76

Releasing the Story from the Tissue

Self-Myofascial Work as Narrative Practice

We have established that the body keeps its own records. That the stories the Monkey tells are not merely mental events — they are held in the tissue, in the chronic patterns of tension and restriction that the fascial web maintains long after the original cause has passed. The grief that collapsed the chest. The unresolved threat that never released from the psoas. The decades of carrying responsibility that turned to stone in the upper trapezius. The feet, walking through a life they were never fully present to. This chapter is about working directly with that stored material. Not through clinical intervention — that requires a trained practitioner's hands and years of palpatory sensitivity — but through what you can reach from the inside, with patience, with presence, and with the right quality of attention. I want to be clear about what this is and is not before we begin. This is not wellness maintenance. This is not self-care in the sense the wellness industry means it – a reward for the week's effort, a treat for the body. When you apply sustained pressure to a restricted area of your own fascia and hold the breath steady through the discomfort and feel the tissue slowly release, you are not pampering yourself. You are interrupting a story that has been running in your body, sometimes for years. You are giving the Monkey's somatic correlate a chance to update. That requires the same quality of direct, patient, non-narrating attention that the previous two chapters have been training. The breath is the foundation. Un-Naming is the companion. What follows is the territory they open into.

The One Principle That Changes Everything

Most people's instinct about releasing tension is to push harder. To force the tissue into compliance. To override the restriction with sufficient intensity. This is how we approach most physical problems – more effort, more pressure, more determination. The fascia does not respond to this. Or rather, it responds briefly — the tissue yields to acute force the way a rubber band yields when pulled, and then returns, usually within hours, to exactly its previous state. Because the force reached the muscle, not the fascia. And it did not reach the story. Fascia responds to low load applied over a long duration. This is its viscoelastic nature: under sustained, gentle pressure, the ground substance — the hydrated gel that fills the spaces between the collagen fibres — gradually shifts its viscosity. It becomes more fluid. The fibres can move relative to each other. The restriction releases. And crucially, this release happens slowly enough that the nervous system can register it — can update its predictive model of what this area is doing, can revise the chronic prediction of tension and threat that has been maintaining the pattern. This is what I call the Fascial Melt. Find the barrier — the first edge of resistance, well before pain. Stop there. Breathe into it with the LSD rhythm from Chapter 12. Hold for a minimum of ninety seconds, and preferably considerably longer. Feel for the gradual softening — not a dramatic pop or snap, but a slow, spreading warmth, a sense of the tissue yielding not to force but to time. Then wait a little longer. The release continues after you think it has finished. The tools that make this accessible at home are simple: a tennis ball, a lacrosse ball, or a fascia roller. No equipment beyond this is necessary. A tennis ball offers softer, more yielding contact — suitable for the feet, the chest, and any area where the tissue is sensitive or the restriction is close to the surface. A lacrosse ball or firm massage ball provides more specific pressure for deeper areas — the upper back, the gluteals, the sides of the hips. A fascia roller covers broader areas and is particularly effective along the posterior chain. None of these are prescriptions. They are suggestions for how to arrive at the tissue's barrier and wait there. The tool is not the practice. The quality of attention you bring to the tool is the practice. The companion to the Fascial Melt is Un-Naming, exactly as described in Chapter 12. Rather than labelling what you feel as tightness or discomfort, stay with the raw quality of the sensation and follow it. Notice when it shifts. Notice the moment the tissue releases — because it is accompanied by a change that is unmistakable when you are genuinely paying attention. A spreading. A softening. Sometimes a warmth. Sometimes, in areas where a significant story is held, something more — a shift in emotional state, a sudden loosening of something that was not obviously connected to the area being worked. This is EMFT in reverse. The tissue releasing the story.

Where the Stories Live: A Map of the Body's Archive

Twenty years of clinical work has given me a strong sense of where stories tend to concentrate. I offer what follows not as a rigid system but as a map – remembering always that the map is not the territory, and that your own body's record is more accurate than any generalisation I can provide. Begin where you are drawn. Return to what genuinely opens something in you.

The Diaphragm and Solar Plexus: The Architecture of Stress

The diaphragm holds the stories of sustained stress – the chronic bracing against a world that feels threatening, the breath that has been held at half-capacity for years without the Monkey noticing. When the diaphragm is restricted, breathing is shallow, the vagus nerve is under-stimulated, and the Monkey's stress narrative has a permanent physiological anchor. The organism is perpetually in a state of mild preparation. Ready for something that never quite arrives. Releasing the diaphragm is one of the most direct routes to parasympathetic activation available outside of clinical treatment. Lie on your back, knees bent, feet flat on the floor. Place the fingertips gently beneath the lower ribs on both sides — not pressing in, simply making contact and waiting. On the exhale, allow the fingertips to follow the ribs inward and upward very slightly, as the diaphragm ascends. Maintain that gentle contact through the next inhale, feeling the ribs expand against your fingers. Stay for several breath cycles. You are not stretching anything. You are reminding the tissue that movement is available here. That there is space. A tennis ball placed beneath the mid-thoracic spine — between the shoulder blades, with the knees bent and the feet flat — can reach the fascial connections of the posterior diaphragm in a way that fingertip contact cannot. Lie onto it rather than rolling. Find the point of greatest density and anchor there. Breathe. The release will arrive in its own time.

The Psoas: The Body's Unfinished Business

The psoas and the Deep Front Line hold the stories of unresolved threat — the sustained vigilance of a nervous system that has never been given clear permission to stand down. The chronic fight-or-flight response that was activated but never completed. The long tension of a life spent preparing for something difficult. The psoas is the deepest hip flexor in the body, running from the lumbar vertebrae through the pelvis to the top of the femur. It is the only muscle that connects the spine directly to the leg. When it is chronically shortened — which it is in almost everyone who sits for extended periods, and in many people who have lived through sustained stress or trauma — it pulls the lumbar spine forward, compresses the sacrum, restricts the breath, and maintains a biological posture that the Monkey narrates as: something is wrong. Something requires vigilance. I must stay ready. A sustained lunge position reaches the psoas where most stretches cannot. The rear knee on the floor, the front shin vertical, the torso upright. Hold for three to five minutes — not thirty seconds, not two minutes, but long enough for the viscoelastic creep to begin. Breathe slowly and completely into the front of the rear hip. Do not lean into the stretch. Simply arrive at the barrier and remain there. The psoas releases in its own time, and when it does, the shift is felt throughout the whole organism — a quality of spaciousness in the lower back and pelvis that those who carry chronic tension there will recognise immediately as unfamiliar.

The Upper Trapezius and Posterior Neck: The Weight of What We Carry

The upper trapezius and posterior neck hold the stories of carrying – of responsibility, of the Monkey's perpetual agenda, of the weight of everything that must be managed and maintained and held together. The shoulders that never fully descend. The neck that never releases its forward tilt. These are among the most universal restriction patterns in modern bodies, and among the most stubbornly maintained, because the story that created them – I carry this, I must keep carrying this – tends to be one the Monkey has deeply identified with. A firm ball against a wall is the most accessible self-treatment for this area. Place a lacrosse ball or tennis ball between the upper trapezius and the wall – roughly between the top of the shoulder and the base of the neck. Apply body weight gently by leaning back into the ball. Find a point of density and stop. Do not roll. This is crucial. Rolling tells the nervous system that the pressure is temporary and passing; the tissue simply waits for it to move on. Anchoring – finding the restriction, arriving, and staying – is what creates the conditions for the Fascial Melt. Hold for sixty to ninety seconds per point. Breathe. When the density softens, move to the adjacent area. The same ball placed between the medial border of the shoulder blade and the spine reaches the deep fascial layers of the posterior thorax — an area that holds, in many people, the accumulated weight of years of desk posture, of bracing, of the subtle but constant muscular effort of holding the world at arm's length. Lie on it rather than standing. Let gravity provide the load. Breathe slowly and allow the tissue time to respond. The quality of attention here matters as much as the position. This is not rolling. This is arriving, staying, and listening.

The Soles of the Feet: Contact with the Ground

The soles of the feet hold something that surprised me when I first paid attention to it: the accumulated story of contact with the ground. Or, more precisely, the story of the absence of that contact — the lifelong habit of walking through the world without actually arriving in it. Feet encased in shoes since childhood, never permitted to feel the surface they stand on, never fully engaged with the proprioceptive information they were designed to gather and transmit. The plantar fascia is the beginning of the Superficial Back Line — the fascial continuity that runs from the soles of the feet up the back of the legs, along the spine, and over the skull to the forehead. What is held in the feet is not local. It ripples upward through the entire posterior chain. Chronic plantar restriction changes the tension of the calves, the hamstrings, the lumbar fascia. The feet are the foundation of the whole structure, and most people have never consciously attended to them. A tennis ball is the right tool here — firm enough to reach the plantar fascia, yielding enough not to overwhelm it. Stand on it, barefoot, with enough body weight to feel the pressure without pain. Begin at the heel and move slowly — not rolling continuously, but moving from point to point, pausing wherever the tissue feels dense or restricted, staying for thirty to sixty seconds before advancing. Cross the arch. Reach the ball of the foot. Work each foot for several minutes before moving to the other. What you are likely to notice, when you first do this attentively, is how much information the soles of your feet contain. Areas of density you were not aware of. Asymmetries between left and right. The particular quality of tissue that has been protected from contact for years. You are not just releasing plantar fascia. You are restoring the body's primary interface with the ground —

reconnecting the Superficial Back Line from its foundation.

The Release and What Follows

I want to prepare you for something that many people find disorienting the first time it happens: a significant fascial release can be accompanied by a sudden shift in emotional state that seems entirely disproportionate to what you were doing physically. Tears arriving from nowhere. A wave of something that is not quite fear and not quite sadness but needs to move through. A sudden, unexpected quality of lightness where there had been nothing but familiar heaviness. This is not unusual. It is EMFT working in the direction of release rather than accumulation. The tissue had been holding a story. The story is leaving. What you are feeling is the story in motion — not stuck, not fixed, not filed, but finally moving through the system as it always needed to. This is the physiology working correctly. Allow it to move. The breath is the guide: keep it slow, steady, and nasal even as the emotion rises. It will pass. Something more spacious arrives after. This spaciousness is not just emotional — it is a genuine change in the tissue, in the quality of the fascial web, in the nervous system's model of what this area of the body is doing. The update has been received. If significant emotional material arises during this work, do not push further into the physical technique. Put the ball or roller aside. Lie flat. Breathe. Use the Un-Naming practice to meet what is arising without immediately labelling or managing it. The tissue has done what it needed to do. What follows is the nervous system integrating the update — and that integration requires time and space, not more intervention. This time is not wasted. It is the work continuing at a depth that the hands cannot reach.

The Sequence That Isn't

The Monkey, at this point, will want a sequence. A clear protocol. A numbered list of exactly what to do and in what order, so that the practice can be performed correctly and evaluated against a standard. I understand this. The Monkey is trying to be helpful. It wants to ensure you get the maximum benefit, to optimise the process, to know when you have done enough. But a fixed sequence is precisely the wrong relationship to have with this practice. A protocol tells the nervous system what is going to happen next, which means the nervous system is already predicting and bracing rather than listening and responding. The restriction you need most on a given day is the one the sequence may not reach until step four, by which point the available time has been used and the Monkey has begun planning the rest of the day. Begin instead with a few minutes of LSD breathing – enough to establish the parasympathetic baseline that the tissue needs in order to release at all. Then simply ask: where is the Monkey holding on today? You will know. The body has been reporting this continuously. You have simply been filtering the signal. Bring the ball or roller to that area. Arrive. Stay. Breathe. Wait for the release, and then – this is the part that cannot be scheduled – wait a little longer. Move when the tissue invites movement, not when the clock says it is time. Your own body will tell you, session by session, where more attention is needed and where the work is complete. This is not a vague instruction. It is the most precise instruction available, because no generalisation I can offer is more accurate than the proprioceptive intelligence already present in the tissue you are working with. Three areas in a single session is usually sufficient. More than that, and you risk opening more than the nervous system can integrate in one sitting. The goal is not to cover ground. The goal is to create the conditions for a genuine update – and then to give the system time and space to receive it.

What the body knew:

The body does not store stories as abstractions. It stores them as physical patterns — fascial restrictions, altered tension, compressed spaces where fluid has ceased to move freely. Releasing those patterns is not merely physical maintenance. It is the practice of intellectual honesty applied to the tissue. It is asking the body: what are you actually holding here? And then — with patience, with presence, without forcing — allowing the honest answer to emerge.

Chapter 14

"The Dao is like a deep well, never overflowing, never exhausted. Everything springs from it and returns again."

— Daodejing, Chapter 4

Entering the Flow

The Practice of Boundlessness

Everything in this book has been preparation for this chapter. And this chapter cannot give you what it is pointing toward. Let me explain that apparent contradiction before we go further. The state that Newberg documented — parietal quieting, DMN deactivation, the dissolution of the self-other boundary — cannot be directly produced by technique. This is not because it is supernatural or reserved for the spiritually advanced. It is because the state, by definition, involves the temporary suspension of the very apparatus that is trying to produce it. The Monkey cannot engineer the Monkey's own silence. The technique cannot dissolve the technician. What practice can do — what the breathing, the Un-Naming, and the self-myofascial work have been preparing the organism for — is create the conditions under which the silence becomes more available. To use the river as the Daodejing uses it: the river does not force its way to the sea. It follows the path of least resistance, yielding to what is, and by yielding, it arrives. Practice is not forcing the arrival. It is removing the obstacles to the natural flow. With that said — let us talk about what actually works.

Meditation: Sitting with the Gap

I have been meditating seriously long before the experiences in summer of 2022 which I described in Chapter 5,, with increasing depth and frequency as the years have passed. I want to share what I have actually found, rather than what the tradition says should happen. The first thing I found was that the Monkey is far louder in the silence than it is in the noise of daily life. The moment I sat and closed my eyes, the commentary intensified. Plans, memories, assessments, self-criticisms, sudden urgent tasks — the Monkey, deprived of external stimulation to narrate, turned its attention inward with enormous energy. This is normal. It is what the DMN does when it is freed from external task-engagement. It is not a sign of failure or an unsuitable mind. It is the beginning. The second thing I found was that the instruction to "clear the mind" is both wrong and, for most beginners, counterproductive. The mind does not clear. The Monkey does not stop. The practice is not the production of silence but the development of a particular relationship to the noise – an ability to observe the commentary without being carried by it. To notice the thought, without adding the next thought to it. The third thing – which arrived more slowly, after months of regular practice – was that the commentary began to develop gaps. Not long ones, initially. A second or two of genuine quiet between the Monkey's sentences. But those gaps had a quality that was unmistakable: a sense of presence, of aliveness, of direct contact with the present moment that the narrative had been obscuring. And in those gaps, sometimes – not always, not reliably, but often enough to reorient everything – something larger became briefly available. The boundlessness. The felt sense of the self-other boundary becoming permeable. What I wrote in my journal as feeling more real than reality. I will not prescribe a specific meditation tradition. There are many, and each has genuine value. What I will offer is the quality of attention that, in my experience, opens the gaps most reliably.

PRACTICE: *The Gap Practice – A Simple Meditation*

Sit comfortably, spine upright but not rigid or lie down if sitting is uncomfortable to you. Eyes closed or softly downcast. Establish the LSD breath: Light, Slow, Deep, through the nose. Let the breath settle for two to three minutes before anything else. Bring attention to the breath itself – not as a technique to be performed, but as a living event happening in the body. The physical sensation of air moving. The rise and fall of the belly. The slight pause between the exhale and the next inhale. When thoughts arise – and they will – do not fight them. Do not follow them into their content. Simply note: thinking. And return to the breath. Not with frustration. With the same patient curiosity you would bring to a physical sensation in the Un-Naming practice. As the session deepens, the gaps between thoughts will lengthen. When a gap arrives, do not name it or reach toward it. Simply rest in it, for as long as it lasts. The gap will close. The Monkey will return. This is not failure. Return to the breath. The next gap will come. Begin with 10 to 20 minutes daily. Over weeks and months, extend to 45 or 60 minutes if possible. The depth of experience is not proportional to the time – but the time creates the conditions in which depth becomes available. One note on expectation: some sessions will be almost entirely Monkey. This is not wasted time. The act of returning – of sitting with the noise without being swept away by it – is itself the practice of being in the territory.

Movement as Meditation: The Qigong Principle

Not everyone finds stillness the easiest gateway. For some bodies – particularly those carrying significant chronic tension, or those whose Monkey is particularly activated by the absence of external stimulus – movement is the more accessible entry point. Qigong – the ancient Chinese practice of coordinated movement, breath, and attention – is not exercise in the conventional sense. Its purpose is not to strengthen muscles or improve cardiovascular fitness, though these can be side effects. Its purpose is to cultivate what practitioners call Qi – which I understand, in the framework of this book, as the free and unobstructed flow of biological process through the liquid matrix of the fascial web. When the tissue is restricted and the breath is shallow and the nervous system is in chronic sympathetic activation, Qi does not flow. The organism is, in the most literal sense, not flowing. The core instruction of Qigong is simple enough to state and demanding enough to practise: every movement is coordinated with the breath, every breath is slow and nasal, and the quality of attention is the same Un-Naming quality that we have been cultivating – present, curious, non-evaluative. The movement is not performed. It is inhabited. When movement is inhabited in this way – when the attention is fully in the body, following the sensation rather than narrating it – something begins to happen that those who have experienced it recognise immediately. The Monkey quiets. Not because it has been suppressed, but because the body's attention is so full that the narrative circuits do not have their usual purchase. This is the flow state described by Csikszentmihalyi – the state in which self-consciousness disappears and the action and the actor become, briefly, one. This is Wu Wei made embodied. Not philosophical non-interference, but the living experience of an organism moving in accord with its own nature, without the friction of a Monkey that is simultaneously trying to manage, evaluate, and narrate the movement. You do not need to learn a specific Qigong form to access this. The principle can be applied to walking – slow walking, conscious walking, walking in which each step is felt rather than thought. To swimming, to cycling, to dancing. To any form of movement that you know well enough that the technique does not require conscious effort, and that you are willing to inhabit rather than perform. The question to ask of any movement practice: am I doing this, or is it happening? The answer, when you are genuinely in the flow, is always both: you become the happening. And the boundary between the two has temporarily dissolved.

What Arrives in the Silence

I want to return, briefly and honestly, to the experiences I described in Chapter 5 — the meditation journal entries, the sense of boundlessness, the colours and the expansion, the all-encompassing love and absolute peace. I described these as neurological events. As the parietal lobes going quiet. As the dissolution of the self-other boundary that Newberg has documented and that consistent meditation practice can produce. All of this is accurate, as far as I can tell. But there is something that the neurological description does not fully capture, and intellectual honesty requires me to say so. The experience of boundlessness, when it comes, does not feel like a neurological event. It feels like contact with something that was always there — something that the ordinary sense of a separate self had been obscuring. Not a new discovery, but a recognition. A returning to something that was, in some sense, always already home. Is this the Dao? Is it the organism briefly perceiving its own fundamental nature? Is it the hard problem becoming briefly transparent — the felt sense of existence before the Monkey builds a story around it? I do not know. I am genuinely uncertain. And I have come to believe that the uncertainty itself — held without panic, without the urgent need for a story to fill it — is part of the practice. What I do know is this: the experience changes things. Not in a dramatic, sudden way. But quietly, over time, the encounters with the silence begin to alter the Monkey's relationship to its own stories. They feel less permanent. Less absolute. The category "this is who I am" loosens slightly. The category "this is how things must be" softens slightly. Not because the Monkey has been defeated, but because it has briefly glimpsed the territory beyond its own maps, and the glimpse, however brief, leaves something behind. The river knows the sea. Even when it cannot see it.

The Practice of Not Arriving

I want to close this chapter with a word of caution that is also a word of encouragement.

The Monkey, as I said at the beginning of Part Three, will attempt to turn the practices of Part Three into a project. A goal. A measure of progress. It will evaluate your meditation sessions as good or bad. It will compare your experiences of flow to the accounts in books and find yours wanting, or it will construct a story of spiritual development in which you are tracking toward enlightenment and the graph is gratifyingly upward. All of this is the Monkey doing what it does. Notice it. Set it gently aside. Return to the breath. The practices in this book are not a path to a destination. They are a way of travelling differently. The territory is not somewhere you are going. It is where you already are, beneath the map. The practice is simply the ongoing, patient, humble work of remembering this – of returning, again and again, from the story to the sensation, from the label to the living experience, from the noise to the gaps between the noise. Every return is complete in itself. There is nowhere to arrive. The Dao follows what is.

What the body knew:

The state that the practices point toward is not a reward for sufficient effort. It is what is already present when the Monkey's effort ceases. The practices do not produce the silence. They remove, gradually and honestly, the habits that prevent the silence from being noticed. The river does not work to reach the sea. It simply flows, and the sea is already at the end of every flow.

Epilogue

"To know not to know is wisdom.
To not know not to know is a flaw.
Recognizing this flaw is the first step to change."
– Daodejing, Chapter 71

The Honest Silence

We have arrived at the place where the map runs out. I have been honest with you throughout this book – about the neuroscience of the Storytelling Monkey, about the hard problem that the neuroscience does not resolve, about the physiological reality of the mystical state, about the stories I have told myself and the stories I have been told by the tissue of the people who have trusted me with their bodies. I want to be honest in these final pages too. I do not know why consciousness exists. I do not know whether the boundlessness encountered in deep meditation is a glimpse of some fundamental nature of reality, or a neurological artefact of parietal deactivation, or both simultaneously in a way that makes the distinction meaningless. I do not know whether the soldier in the green uniform carrying the Daodejing was a past life, a confabulation of my own history and longing, or a symbolic figure generated by the Monkey to help me finally let go of something that needed releasing. I know the letting go was real. I know what I felt in the session, and in the weeks and months after it. The cause remains, honestly, uncertain.

I have found, over the years of living with these questions, that the uncertainty itself has become something to rest in rather than flee from. The Monkey still wants answers. It will always want answers — that is what it was built for. But the part of me that has spent time in the territory, however briefly, knows that the absence of an answer is not the same as the absence of meaning. It is, in fact, where meaning lives — not in the story, but in the direct encounter with existence that precedes the story. The hard problem of consciousness has not been solved. It may never be solved, for the reasons we explored in Chapter 6: we are attempting to use consciousness to understand consciousness, to see the eye with the eye. Every framework we build — materialism, panpsychism, integrated information theory, the Dao — is another map. The territory remains beyond the reach of any map. And yet you are reading these words. And there is something it is like to be you, reading them. Something is here, aware, feeling, present. The hard problem is not an abstract philosophical puzzle. It is the most intimate fact of your existence. You are the mystery. This is not a comfortable conclusion. The Monkey wants a resolution. It wants a final answer, a coherent story, a settled metaphysical framework that explains what you are and why you are here. I cannot give you that. Nobody can, honestly. What I can offer is this: the practices in Part Three are not a path to the answer. They are a practice of living honestly with the question. Of being in the gap — not falling into it, not filling it, but dwelling in it with the same equanimity that the Daodejing has always counselled. The Dao follows what is. Not what we wish were the case. Not what the Monkey's story requires. What is. Something has shifted in me in the years of writing this book and the years of practice that preceded it. I do not want to overstate this. The Monkey is still here, doing what it does — narrating, evaluating, planning, sometimes catastrophising. The stories still arise. The tissue still holds its patterns. I am still a human being with the full equipment of a human being, including the full weight of its evolutionary inheritance. But the relationship to all of this has changed. The stories feel less like walls and more like weather. They move through rather than defining the space. The silence between the sentences is more familiar – not comfortable exactly, because genuine silence is too alive to be comfortable in the Monkey's sense of the word, but recognisable. Known. Something I can return to. My patients, over the course of this work, have taught me more than any book. Bodies do not lie. The tissue holds what the mind has stopped consciously acknowledging. And when the tissue releases – when the fascial restriction that held a story for a decade finally yields under sustained, patient, present attention – the intelligence of the organism is available in a form that the Monkey's narrative never quite reaches. Something in the body already knows how to heal. Already knows how to let go. Already knows how to flow. The practice is simply learning to get out of the way. I want to leave you with the image that has accompanied this entire book, and that returns to me most reliably in the moments when the Monkey falls quiet. A river. Not a metaphor for something else. An actual river – the movement of water from higher ground to lower, following the path of least resistance, yielding to every obstacle without losing its direction, wearing away the hardest stone not through force but through presence and time. The river does not try to reach the sea. It simply moves with the nature of water. The sea is the inevitable consequence. You are the river. Not the story of the river that the Monkey tells. The river itself — the actual, moving, present-moment flow of biological process, consciousness, sensation, and life that is happening right now, whether the Monkey is narrating it or not. The sea is already at the end of every flow. You have never been anywhere else.

Put the book down. Breathe. Feel the ground beneath you. The territory is already here.

Steve Brandl

Ho Chi Minh City, Vietnam

References and Further Reading

The following lists the works cited or drawn upon throughout this book, organised by theme, together with a note on how each appears in the argument. Works marked with an asterisk (*) are particularly recommended for readers who wish to go deeper into a specific area.

I. *Consciousness and the Storytelling Monkey*

Seth, A. (2021). Being You: A New Science of Consciousness. Dutton / Faber & Faber. [* Essential. The most accessible and scientifically rigorous account of consciousness as 'controlled hallucination' and the predictive brain. Central to Chapters 1 and 2. Seth engages the hard problem honestly without dismissing it.]

Chalmers, D. (1995). 'Facing Up to the Problem of Consciousness'. Journal of Consciousness Studies, 2(3), pp. 200–219. [* The paper that named the hard problem. Short, readable, and foundational. Central to Chapter 6.]

Goff, P. (2019). Galileo's Error: Foundations for a New Science of Mind. Pantheon Books. [* Argues that science since Galileo deliberately excluded consciousness from its framework, creating the hard problem. Provocative and intellectually honest. Chapter 6.]

Metzinger, T. (2003). Being No One: The Self-Model Theory of Subjectivity. MIT Press. [For the philosophically committed reader. The technical foundation for the phenomenal self-model concept used in Chapter 2.]

Metzinger, T. (2009). The Ego Tunnel: The Science of the Mind and the Myth of the Self. Basic Books. [* More accessible version of the same framework. Recommended for general readers interested in the transparent self-model.]

Gazzaniga, M. S. (1998). The Mind's Past. University of California Press. [The Interpreter and split-brain research. Chapters 1 and 2.]

McGilchrist, I. (2009). The Master and His Emissary: The Divided Brain and the Making of the Western World. Yale University Press. [* The left-hemisphere Interpreter as curator with an agenda. Chapter 2. A profound and demanding work.]

Frankish, K. (2016). 'Illusionism as a Theory of Consciousness'. Journal of Consciousness Studies, 23(11–12), pp. 11–39. [The illusionist position on the hard problem. Chapter 6.]

Tononi, G. (2008). 'Consciousness as Integrated Information: A Provisional Manifesto'. Biological Bulletin, 215(3), pp. 216–242. [Integrated Information Theory and the distributed nature of consciousness. Chapter 6.]

Friston, K. (2010). 'The Free-Energy Principle: A Unified Brain Theory?'. Nature Reviews Neuroscience, 11(2), pp. 127–138. [Active inference and predictive processing. For technically inclined readers. Background to Chapters 1 and 2.]

Clark, A. (2023). The Experience Machine: How Our Minds Predict and Shape Reality. Pantheon Books. [* Accessible account of predictive processing. Recommended as a companion to Seth for readers who want the full picture without the technical papers.]

II. The Body, Fascia, and Emotional Myofascial Tension

van der Kolk, B. (2014). The Body Keeps the Score: Brain, Mind, and Body in the Healing of Trauma. Viking / Penguin. [* The foundational text on trauma stored in the body. This book extends van der Kolk's argument beyond traumatic experience to all narrative identity. Chapters 3 and 9.]

Damasio, A. (1999). The Feeling of What Happens: Body and Emotion in the Making of Consciousness. Harcourt Brace. [* Somatic marker hypothesis: emotion and feeling as the foundation of consciousness, not an add-on. Validates the EMFT concept with serious neuroscience. Chapter 3.]

Porges, S. W. (2011). The Polyvagal Theory: Neurophysiological Foundations of Emotions, Attachment, Communication, and Self-Regulation. W. W. Norton. [* The vagus nerve as the body's calm highway. Polyvagal Theory and its implications for fascial health, breathing, and emotional regulation. Chapters 10 and 12.]

Levine, P. A. (1997). Waking the Tiger: Healing Trauma. North Atlantic Books. [Somatic experiencing and the body's completion of thwarted threat responses. Background to the EMFT concept.]

Brandl, S. (2024). Fascia-Puncture: Transforming Health from Within. Self-published. [The clinical foundation for the EMFT concept and the Fascial Melt technique. The present book extends and reframes the work developed there.]

III. Pain, Narrative, and the Limits of the Predictive Model

Gordon, A. and Ziv, A. (2021). The Way Out: A Revolutionary, Scientifically Proven Approach to Healing Chronic Pain. Avery / Penguin Random House. [* Pain Reprocessing Therapy and the neuroscience of story-change. The 2021 JAMA Psychiatry trial validation. Chapter 9. Recommended for anyone living with chronic pain.]

Ashar, Y. K., Gordon, A., Schubiner, H. et al. (2021). 'Effect of Pain Reprocessing Therapy vs Placebo and Usual Care for Patients With Chronic Back Pain: A Randomized Clinical Trial'. JAMA Psychiatry, 79(1), pp. 13–23. [The clinical trial underlying Gordon and Ziv's book. For readers who want the peer-reviewed evidence.]

IV. *Mystical Experience, Flow, and the Neuroscience of Oneness*

Newberg, A. and Waldman, M. R. (2001). Why God Won't Go Away: Brain Science and the Biology of Belief. Ballantine Books. [* Neurotheology: parietal lobe quieting during peak mystical experience. The neural correlates of boundlessness. Chapter 5.]

Csikszentmihalyi, M. (1990). Flow: The Psychology of Optimal Experience. Harper & Row. [* Flow state and the disappearing self. DMN deactivation and effortless action. Chapter 5.]

Brewer, J. A., Worhunsky, P. D., Gray, J. R., et al. (2011). 'Meditation Experience Is Associated with Differences in Default Mode Network Activity and Connectivity'. Proceedings of the National Academy of Sciences, 108(50), pp. 20254–20259. [DMN reduction in experienced meditators. Chapter 2.]

V. *Breathing and the Autonomic Nervous System*

Nestor, J. (2020). Breath: The New Science of a Lost Art. Riverhead Books. [* Comprehensive and accessible account of the science of functional breathing – nasal breathing, the Bohr effect, breath rate and autonomic regulation. Recommended alongside Chapter 12.]

Bohr, C., Hasselbalch, K. and Krogh, A. (1904). 'Ueber einen in biologischer Beziehung wichtigen Einfluss, den die Kohlensäurespannung des Blutes auf dessen Sauerstoffbindung übt'. Skandinavisches Archiv für Physiologie, 16, pp. 402–412. [The original Bohr effect paper. The physiological basis for the LSD breathing principle. Chapter 12.]

VI. *Somatic Practice and Awareness*

Gendlin, E. T. (1978). Focusing. Everett/Edwards. [* The felt sense and the pre-verbal body. Focusing technique as a form of Un-Naming. Chapter 13. Underused and underknown – essential reading for practitioners.]

VII. *Philosophy, Shared Fictions, and the Critique of Dogma*

Laozi (c. 4th century BCE). Daodejing. Various translations; quotations in this book are from the author's own translation found in "From Nothing to Infinity: The Daodejing and the Foundation of Wisdom". [* The most intellectually honest metaphysical framework ever articulated. Epigraph to every chapter. The conceptual spine of the book.]

Zhuangzi (c. 3rd century BCE). Zhuangzi: The Complete Writings. Translated by Brook Ziporyn (2020), Hackett Publishing. [The cook and the ox: flow state and Wu Wei embodied. Chapter 15.]

Harari, Y. N. (2011). Sapiens: A Brief History of Humankind. Harper. [Shared fictions — money, nations, brands — as the Storytelling Monkey's civilisational operating system. Chapter 8.]

Hitchens, C. (2007). God Is Not Great: How Religion Poisons Everything. Twelve / Hachette. [The institutionalisation of mystical experience as dogma. The distinction between felt experience and organised religion. Chapter 4.]

VIII. *The Author's Previous Work*

The present book develops arguments introduced in the following earlier works by Steve Brandl:

Siddhartha and the Storytelling Monkey. Self-published. [The Monkey concept, the Naming Trap, Gazzaniga's Interpreter. The first book in this lineage.]

Fascia-Puncture: Transforming Health from Within. Self-published. [EMFT, LSD breathing, Polyvagal Theory, and the clinical foundation for the Web of Life concept.]

From Nothing to Infinity. Self-published. [Meditation reflections and the Nothing/Infinity framework. Quoted as personal testimony in Chapter 5.]

The Atheist's Jesus. Self-published. [Secular wisdom across traditions and morality without dogma.]

Nothing But the Truth. Self-published. [Subjectivity of experience and the Kara/Ben dialogue framework.]

IX. Resources for Further Practice

For Taijiquan, Breathwork Masterclass and Qigong training, the author recommends:

Taoist Wellness:
taoistwellness.com /
https://www.taoistwellness.online/

For a comprehensive introduction to Qigong theory and practice:

Cohen, K. S. (1997). The Way of Qigong: The Art and Science of Chinese Energy Healing. Ballantine Books. [Comprehensive and scientifically grounded. Recommended for readers wishing to develop a Qigong practice beyond what Chapter 15 can offer.]

Table of Content

www.ingramcontent.com/pod-product-compliance
Lightning Source LLC
LaVergne TN
LVHW090404210926
848480LV00002B/445